Sciatica and Piriformis Syndrome

Sciatica and Piriformis Syndrome

Simple and Effective Exercises for Buttock, Leg and Back Pain

Katharina Brinkmann
Nicolai Napolski

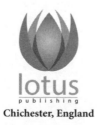

lotus
publishing
Chichester, England

Important note
The content of this book has been researched and carefully verified to the best knowledge and belief of the authors and publisher against sources they consider to be trustworthy. Nevertheless, this book is no substitute for individual fitness and medical advice. For medical advice, please consult a qualified doctor. The publisher and the authors shall not be liable for any negative effects directly or indirectly associated with the information given in this book.

First published by riva Verlag, rivaverlag.de.
This English language edition published in 2017 by
Lotus Publishing
Apple Tree Cottage, Inlands Road, Nutbourne, Chichester, PO18 8RJ

Picture credits: shutterstock/ellepigrafica: p. 10, 13 (upper);
shutterstock/Sebastian Kaulitzki: p. 13 (lower), 14;
squaredotmedia GbR: p. 89 (upper); private: p. 14 (lower)
Exercise photos: squaredotmedia GbR, www.squaredot.media
Editor: Dr Kirsten Reimers
Cover design: Julia Jund, Munich
Cover illustrations: shutterstock/Maridav
Text design: Medlar Publishing Solutions Pvt Ltd., India
Translation: Surrey Translation Services, Woking
Printed and bound in the UK by Short Run Press Limited

British Library Cataloguing-in-Publication Data
A CIP record for this book is available from the British Library
ISBN 978 1 905367 84 9

Contents

Acknowledgements 7

CHAPTER 1
Sciatic Pain 9

CHAPTER 2
Small Piriformis, Big Problem 12

CHAPTER 3
Causes of Piriformis Syndrome 15

CHAPTER 4
Stress and its Effect on Our Minds and Bodies 17

CHAPTER 5
In Practice 21

CHAPTER 6
Releasing Tension 23

CHAPTER 7
Myofascial Relaxation 51

CHAPTER 8
Strengthening the Muscles 58

CHAPTER 9
Sitting Correctly 72

CHAPTER 10
Additional Measures 75

CHAPTER 11
Piriformis Syndrome and Athletes 78

CHAPTER 12
Conscious Movement is the Best Prevention and Therapy 80

Index *89*

About the Authors *93*

Acknowledgements

A big thank you to Dr Torsten Pfitzer for the wonderful expert interview, and to Peter Posner and the sports experts from Trainingsworld, who provided us with advice.

We have started a Facebook group for those affected to share their experiences. You can find us at:

https://www.facebook.com/groups/1702757513312453

'Piriformis syndrome. Helping people help themselves!'

We would be happy to add you to this group so that you can share your experience with us.

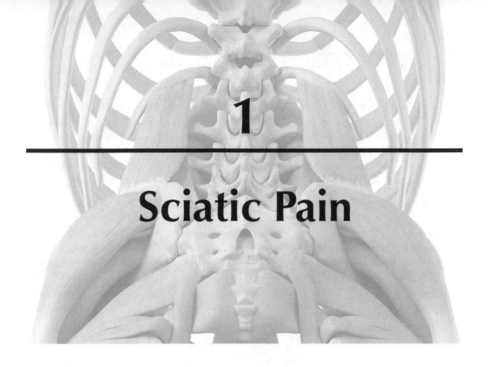

1

Sciatic Pain

A few years ago, while I (Nicolai) was climbing, I felt a strong stabbing pain – like an electric shock – that moved through my left leg, as if from nowhere. I had absolutely no idea what it could have been. What is more, I consider myself reasonably fit and healthy: although I spend at least eight hours per day sitting at a desk in front of my computer, I spend the little free time I have by running as often as possible, and by going climbing from time to time. Having said this, I had just moved to a new flat, and that had been a stressful experience. The first few days after I first felt this pain were torturous – I had severe pains in my buttocks, legs and hips, and could not even think about sitting or walking comfortably.

The diagnosis from my GP was fairly vague: 'Something to do with the sciatic nerve.' The result? Six sessions of physiotherapy, in the hope that the problem would become somehow manageable. I was fortunate enough to see a really great, highly dedicated specialist, who fairly quickly was able to give the correct diagnosis after the appropriate tests: piriformis syndrome.

The *piriformis muscle* is a small, but important, pear-shaped muscle. Together with the sciatic nerve, it runs up and back from the tip of the large femur bone (the greater trochanter, which serves as the base of the muscles in the buttocks), through the large opening in the sit bones (greater sciatic foramen), to the front of the sacral bone. The piriformis crosses the hip and iliosacral joints; it is involved in the outward rotation of the hip joint and the splaying of the thighs, and serves as a flexible pelvic stabiliser.

The *sciatic nerve*, measuring about one finger-width in diameter and also called the *ischiatic nerve*, is the strongest nerve in the human body. It starts in the spinal cord, at the level of the fourth lumbar vertebra to the third sacral vertebra. In many people, the nerve exits the pelvis directly under the piriformis muscle. From there, it continues through the pelvic muscles and over the back of the thigh into the knee joint. It then branches off and sends nerve strands into the foot.

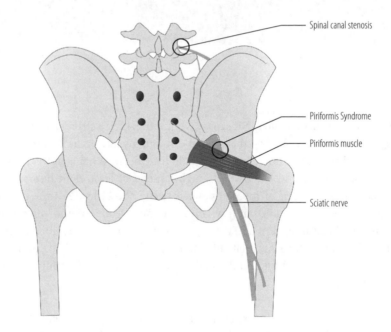

Spinal canal stenosis

Piriformis Syndrome

Piriformis muscle

Sciatic nerve

Thanks to the expert advice of my physiotherapist and to targeted exercises, we were able to get my symptoms of piriformis syndrome under control relatively quickly. After a few weeks, I was – and thankfully have stayed – almost pain-free!

Since then, I have learnt that I am not alone in having this problem: the number of people suffering from this syndrome increases every day! More and more frequently I read that spinal disc surgery could be avoided if piriformis syndrome were clearly diagnosed and treated.

It is impossible to make a generalised judgement on whether a specific group of people is more affected by piriformis syndrome. It is suspected that women are more likely to suffer from it, but ultimately there are no reliable figures or statistics. In older people the causes are often shortened muscles and degenerative changes, while in younger people piriformis syndrome is more often related to sport.

In any case, many people can benefit from this book, from mothers who would just like to be able to play with their children again without pain, to people who sit a lot for their jobs (such as lorry drivers and desk workers) or trained runners who can hardly get out of bed because of pain.

Once you have read this book, you will understand what YOU can do to counteract piriformis syndrome over the long term, or to achieve pain relief with targeted exercises for acute episodes. The material presented within should help you to return to a healthy, pain-free daily routine.

> If you have sciatica-like pain, indicating piriformis syndrome, it is essential to consult a doctor before starting the training programme in this book. If necessary, get a second opinion – consult chiropractors, physiotherapists or osteopaths.

2

Small Piriformis, Big Problem

Statistics show that over 30% of the general population regularly have back problems, but it is not always easy for doctors to determine the underlying causes. There are simply too many conditions that resemble each other – medical textbooks are full of them. For example, piriformis syndrome, a blockage of the sacroiliac joint, tumours or inflammation, polyneuropathy and even lumbago can cause symptoms that overlap with those of a slipped disc.

Physiotherapist Peter Posner summarises the most common diagnoses as follows:

'Lumbar syndrome or lumbosciatica, sometimes lumbar spine syndrome or recurrent lumbago, a previous slipped disc or hernia, perhaps a blockage of the sacroiliac joint or similar …'

Some of these conditions can be remedied with mild pain therapy or corrections to posture, while for others surgery is sometimes necessary. Ultimately, a doctor must decide on the best course of treatment. Try to obtain test results that are as accurate as possible for your pain, and get several opinions if necessary.

Unfortunately, doctors often no longer have the time they need to carry out comprehensive diagnostics, and many people have experienced this. As in my case, patients are often sent to physiotherapists without a concrete diagnosis. Many of them feel abandoned and uncertain.

One of the reasons it is so difficult to diagnose piriformis syndrome is that it cannot be determined with 100% certainty by means of common tests.

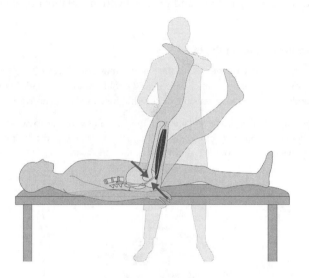

One of the most well-known standard neurological tests is the straight-leg raise. For this, the patient lies on his or her back; the physiotherapist slowly lifts the patient's leg, while the knee is straight, as high as it will go –
up to 90 degrees, where the foot points towards the ceiling. Generally, extension-related pain begins at between 40 and 70 degrees, which may be a sign of sciatic nerve or nerve root inflammation.

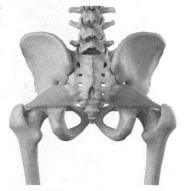

In many cases, this test is then followed by ankle dorsiflexion (Bragard's sign). For this, the patient also lies on his or her back; the physiotherapist again lifts the patient's leg with the knee straight, and the foot is then flexed, so that the toes point towards the head. If the pain radiates from the back towards the thigh, this can be a sign of nerve root inflammation; if the pain occurs in the thigh, this suggests shortened sacroiliac muscles in the pelvic area.

Thus, even when the right diagnosis is made – such as an inflamed piriformis – it is helpful only in rare cases. For long-lasting, successful therapy, it is important to find the cause of the symptoms and proceed with a suitably targeted approach.

The hips – a focal point in the body

The hips determine our symmetry. With their many muscles – over 40 are found in this part of the body – they are our central support and enable us to make various movements: abduction, adduction, flexion, extension, circumduction, and lateral and medial rotations.

However, the hip joint and its cartilage structure are fairly prone to wear. The tiniest differences between your two hip joints can cause an unequal distribution of forces, having a negative effect on your legs and trunk in the long term.

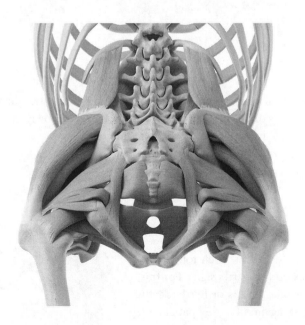

3

Causes of Piriformis Syndrome

Daily Routine – Our Worst Enemy

A fall and repetitive stress, such as sitting for a long time at a desk or in a car, are two of the most common causes of inflammation of the piriformis. If your wallet presses into your buttocks, the inflammation can also be increased; this is because pressure is applied to the muscles and nerves over a long period.

Our bodies are not designed to sit still for extended periods of time. Not so long ago, humans still spent most of their days on their feet, whether hunting, working the fields or completing domestic chores. Consequently, a wide range of demands were placed on the spine, keeping it in constant movement – in all directions.

Today, machines have taken our place in many activities, meaning that we spend much of our time sitting down – both at work and at home – in front of our computers, televisions and smartphones. Our musculoskeletal system wastes away, and the lower back becomes our main point of support; it is only a matter of time until sciatica, piriformis syndrome and back pain occur!

People of all ages can suffer from piriformis syndrome. Such pain can even occur in schoolchildren if chairs are outdated or not appropriate, or if they do not allow individual seating.

Piriformis Syndrome – What Does It Mean?

Simply put, the sciatic nerve passes by the piriformis muscle. If the piriformis is hardened, shortened or inflamed for any of the reasons given above, a notch is created that presses onto the sciatic nerve. Once inflamed, the nerve then radiates the typical sharp stabbing pain into the hips, buttocks and legs. For me, as an example, too much stress, incorrect posture and sitting for long periods of time were the triggers.

According to Alicia Filley, a health and fitness expert, there are other symptoms too. Occasionally, numbness and tingling – like an electric shock – can continue to the calf and toes; severe pain in the knee area can also be experienced. In addition to these symptoms, lower back pain (in the lumbar area) can occur, becoming worse on sitting for long intervals.

As the symptoms of piriformis syndrome can be similar to those of a slipped disc, however, a thorough medical check-up is essential. Nevertheless, keep the following in mind: even if a slipped disc is diagnosed, it may be the case that piriformis syndrome is responsible for your pain, rather than the slipped disc.

Alicia Filley makes reference to an American study in which researchers examined 239 patients with sciatica that was not associated with the intervertebral discs. Many of these patients had previously undergone lumbar spine surgery, as a slipped disc was suspected to be the cause of the pain. However, in most cases this brought no, or very little, relief.

4

Stress and its Effect on Our Minds and Bodies

In the weeks before my injury, I (Nicolai) was under a lot of stress, both physically and mentally, as a result of moving to a new flat. As I was working full-time, I only had the evenings to prepare for the move.

Everything had to be packed up in a very short time. The boxes were much too heavy, and of course I did not think about how to lift them properly and healthily. Most of the time I was eating fast food. On top of all that, my new landlord fell ill and could not be reached a week before the moving date, I still did not have a rental contract, and no one knew where the keys to the new flat were. But I absolutely had to leave the old flat.

It was only with hindsight that I realised that these circumstances had caused my physical and mental health to fall completely out of balance. Studies show that in many cases, pain in the lumbar, thoracic and cervical spines is psychosomatic (in other words, stress-related) pain. Experts think this may be true for up to 85% of cases.

If there is no obvious trauma that could have led to a problem with your piriformis or back, you should ask yourself how much pressure you are under at work and in your private life. Consult a psychotherapist if you think it may help. Once we are aware of the intensity of the pressures we face, stress can be alleviated relatively easily with exercise and relaxation.

Physically, stress can even cause the muscles to harden and shorten as a result of the permanent inner tension. A limited range of motion and incorrect posture are the logical consequences of this.

As physiotherapist Angi Peukert notes, the body is in a vicious circle, as external stress causes internal stress. In addition, each makes the other worse: physical shifts in posture, prolonged periods of illness and financial losses perpetuate the cycle. Pain becomes chronic, and our 'pain memory' is activated; this records very intense pain, as the emotional self is also under great strain. As a result, this pain can occur again whenever another stressful situation is encountered.

To escape from the vicious circle, you can take action in various ways with changes to your diet, your sleep patterns and physical exercise. The second part of this book takes a closer look at the third aspect, but first we will briefly cover the first two: eating and sleeping.

Food

A poor diet can have a very significant impact on the health of your muscles. One of the main causes of pain is inflammation; not only can this occur as a result of overexertion, poor posture and other physical problems, but also stress, environmental toxins and a poor diet can be responsible. In principle, acute inflammation is a reasonable consequence, because this is how our body reacts to injuries: it sends its 'helpers' to repair the damage. However, when inflammation becomes chronic, we end up in a sort of 'crisis mode'; this crisis mode is encouraged by a poor diet and environmental toxins, such as chemicals and pesticides, among other things.

Carbohydrates in sugar and wheat, and even wholemeal bread with a high glycaemic index, are some of the biggest triggers and promoters of chronic inflammation. High blood sugar and insulin levels cause the body to constantly be in crisis mode. Studies show that refined sugar, processed flour, vegetable oils and many other ingredients found in industrially processed foods are to a large extent responsible for inflammatory conditions.

This means it is best to avoid the following:

- Gluten-free products with high sugar and grain content.
- Industrially processed foods: white flour and products made from it, white rice, conventional ready meals, sausages and meat products with nitrates, standard protein and energy bars.
- Meat that is overcooked.
- Industrial vegetable oils with an unhealthy ratio of omega-3 to omega-6 fatty acids.

In order to combat inflammation, it is advisable to eat more organic and sustainable products with high antioxidant effects, such as:

- Bone broth.
- Vegetables: bean sprouts, spinach, garlic, broccoli, red cabbage, green cabbage, spring onions, chard, olives, tomatoes, courgettes, onions.
- Fruit: apples, avocados, pears, cherries, mandarins, oranges, papayas, peaches, lemons.
- Berries: raspberries, blackberries, cranberries, strawberries, blueberries.
- Fish: halibut, herring, cod, mackerel, salmon, trout, whitefish, tuna (please keep to organic, sustainable varieties, ideally wild-caught).
- Nuts and seeds: walnuts, pecans, peanuts, chestnuts, sunflower seeds.
- Coconut oil, virgin olive oil.
- Herbs and spices: turmeric, red pepper, ginger, oregano.
- Green tea, ginger tea.
- Red wine (no more than one glass per day).

Sleep

We have known for a long time the importance of a good night's sleep. Unfortunately, our daily lives have become very fast-paced, and we also spend too much time in front of televisions, smartphones and tablets late at night. With their bright light and almost imperceptible flickering, screens are a source of constant stimulation, making it very difficult for us to 'switch off'.

To really be relaxed and rejuvenated, we need at least seven hours of sleep – the hours of sleep before midnight are the ones that count the most! It is therefore essential to optimise your deep sleep: try to go to bed before 11 pm and avoid using digital devices after 10 pm. The darker your bedroom, the better. Always switch off the internet and other electronic devices – including your smartphone.

On the Path to a Pain-free Life

Before we move on to the second part of the book – the exercises – here is one more tip for you. Get to know your body and how it works as a whole, accept your injury and always keep some key points in mind:

- Be physically active.
- Avoid lifting incorrectly and with poor posture.
- Try to reduce your stress levels as much as possible.
- Think about getting enough deep sleep.
- Do not forget your diet.
- Make sure to sit with a straight back.
- Most importantly: try to get an exact diagnosis of your problem. Be willing to seek out several opinions!

Hopefully you will then be back on the path to a pain-free life. We wish you all the best!

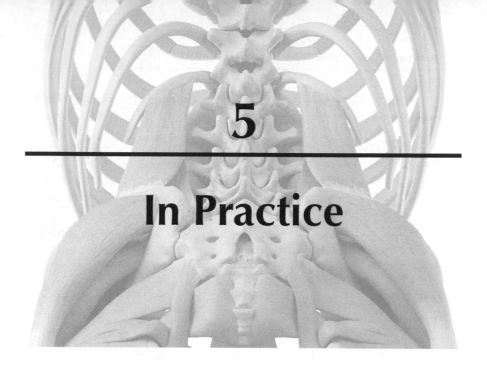

5

In Practice

The good news? Pain in the buttocks, indicating piriformis syndrome, is not irreparable: you can do something about it! Mobilising movements for the pelvis and hips stimulate the metabolism and accelerate your recovery. That being the case, do not just put your feet up and wait for your condition to get better by itself.

In the chapters in this part of the book, we will introduce you to exercises and techniques for prevention – but that also relieve pain in critical cases.

During acute episodes of pain, choose exercises primarily from the 'Releasing Tension' chapter. The localised stretches and myofascial relaxation for the piriformis will quickly provide relief. The next step is to remain pain-free over the long term. This takes the form of regular stretching of the piriformis and all the muscles around the hip area. Strength training is also important for combating the consequences of overexertion.

First of all, however, look for the causes. In most cases, piriformis syndrome cannot be attributed to obvious causes, such as a fall: usually, it is related to posture and stress. In order to be pain-free over the long term, and remain so, it is therefore important to look at the underlying causes.

Why stretching alone does not help

While stretching exercises do indeed help to release tension, their success is generally only short-lived, since you target the symptom, not the cause, with these exercises. The muscle stays weak, and daily stresses mean that the tension quickly returns.

Why? Muscles tense because they are overworked by overexertion, incorrect use and poor posture. The piriformis muscle and the neighbouring muscles can no longer do their job and subsequently 'resign'. This is why it is important to strengthen the muscles for the long term, so that they can work better.

6

Releasing Tension

Localised Stretching for the Piriformis

We begin with stretching exercises that are specifically adapted to the piriformis muscle. In acute cases, these are very good for relieving pain, and are recommended on days spent mostly sitting, as they relax the buttocks.

The exercises also reach the muscles closer to the surface of the buttocks. The two muscle groups are found right next to each other, and to a large extent play similar roles.

Recommendations for Stretching

How long should I stay in the stretch?
The piriformis is a hip stabiliser, located deep in the body, that provides consistent support to keep the body upright. For this reason, *stretches must be held for at least one minute* – or even a little longer.

Which stretching methods should I use?

We recommend *passive stretching*. This means that you remain in one position for a certain length of time (at least 60 seconds), and you use your own bodyweight, gravity and the interactions between muscles to produce tensile stress. Holding a fixed position also brings the connective tissue into the stretch.

Should I only stretch the painful side?

For each exercise, switch to the other side too. All exercises are designed to be carried out on both sides. As you stretch, keep your full awareness in the moment and take note of any differences between left and right sides.

The piriformis and gluteus maximus muscles

The 'large' gluteus muscle and the 'small' piriformis are good friends. Unfortunately, however, the larger of the two is often weakened and tends to be lazy. In this case, the smaller one – the piriformis – not only provides movement but also ensures our stability, working on behalf of the larger one.

Lying on Your Back

Stretching while lying on your back is particularly comfortable and good for pain relief, as you do not have to struggle with balance or an upright posture. You can surrender yourself to gravity and enjoy the stretch for longer.

Knee to Opposite Shoulder

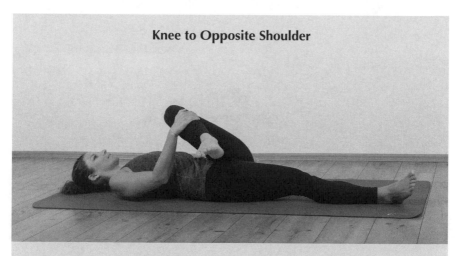

This exercise specifically targets the piriformis. The thigh is subjected to adduction and an internal rotation.

- Bend your left leg and pull it up towards your upper body. The knee forms a right angle. The right leg remains straight on the mat; alternatively, you can place your right foot near your buttocks, to release the strain on the lower back.
- Hold your left knee with your right hand and pull it towards your right shoulder. Keep the knee at a 90-degree angle.
- The left buttock and shoulders remain on the mat.

How do I reach the piriformis?

Any movement of the hips reaches the piriformis to some degree. The piriformis is a short, strong external rotator, and a rather weaker abductor when the hips are moved. In other words, it works when you turn your leg outwards, away from your body – this is called *external rotation*. Think of a ballet dancer, or Charlie Chaplin. In addition to its main role in external rotation, the muscle also supports abduction, the splaying of the legs outwards.

If we want to stretch the piriformis, we have to go against its 'working direction' in order to bring length to the muscle.

Because of the role of the piriformis as a strong external rotator, it is important to use an internal rotation of the thigh and hip to fully stretch the muscle (see above). Hip movements in combination with an external rotation have an optimal effect on the muscles in the buttocks (see 'Leg Knotting' exercise, p. 26). A combination of both of these stretches, for the piriformis and the buttocks, gives the best results.

Leg Knotting

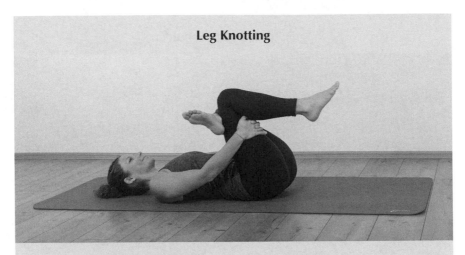

- Place both feet near your buttocks. Place the outside of your left ankle on your right thigh. Your left knee should point outwards.
- Hold the back of your right thigh with both hands and pull your right leg towards your upper body as far as is comfortable. You should feel a pleasant stretch in the muscles on the left side of your buttocks.
- While pulling your thigh in, slide your sit bones down and away and press your lower back into the mat.
- Now pull your right thigh a little further to the left to really target the piriformis (see 'How do I reach the piriformis?', p. 25).
- Remember to keep your head and shoulders relaxed on the mat.

▷ **Tip:** *If you cannot yet reach your thigh, try this variation:*

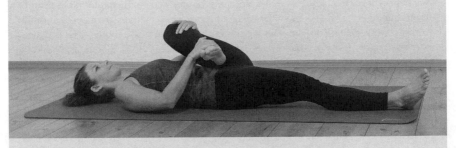

- Hold your left knee with your left hand, and your left ankle with your right hand.
- Pull your lower leg diagonally towards you – as far as is comfortable for you.
- Pull the leg a little further to the right to really get to your piriformis.

Knee-down Twist

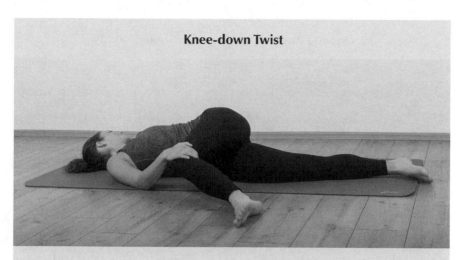

- Bend your left leg and pull it up towards your upper body. The other leg stays straight on the mat.
- With your right hand, hold the outside of your left knee. Gently pull your left knee to the right side and place it on the floor or on a cushion. Lift the buttocks slightly and turn your pelvis a little to the right.
- Stretch your left arm out to the side and turn your upper body to the left. Push your left shoulder towards the mat.
- Your ribs on the left side sink down and to the left. Direct all of your attention to this area and sink further and further.

▷ **Tip:** *Keep your bottom leg straight so that you can move your top leg further down and potentially rotate it further inwards. This allows you to reach the piriformis, etc. better.*

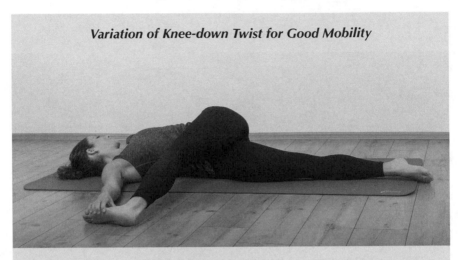

Variation of Knee-down Twist for Good Mobility

- Hold your foot with the opposite hand and stretch your leg to the side.

For this variation, your back leg muscles should be fairly flexible, as this is an intense stretch for the thigh as well as the piriformis. Tightness of the muscles in this area – i.e. the hamstrings – can lead to incorrect posture in the pelvis and reinforce curvature of the lower back.

Sitting

Seated stretching exercises are effective and intense, as you work in forward fold (see p. 32) a great deal. For lying poses, you can achieve a similar effect by raising your legs – this moves the hips. Compared with the lying position, the effects of gravity and the weight of the upper body are stronger when you are sitting.

Sitting Half Spinal Twist

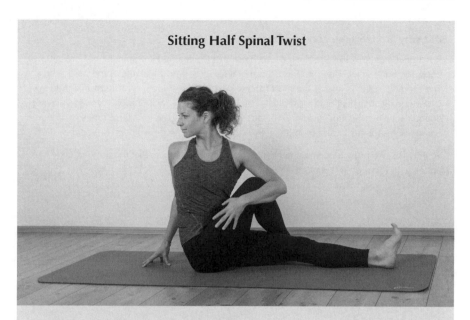

This stretch targets the posterior hip muscles.

- Sit on the floor with your legs out in front of you. Bend your right leg and place it over your left leg so that your right foot is about level with your left knee.
- Hold your right knee with both hands and bring length to your spine. Consciously align yourself. When sitting upright, you should feel both sit bones in contact with the floor. If this is not the case, you can practise the sitting half spinal twist on a cushion to make it easier for you to sit upright.
- Move your left elbow or hand to the right knee and twist your upper body to the right, keeping it upright. The right knee presses into the left armpit. Support yourself with your right hand behind your buttocks.
- Relax both shoulders.
- In this position, the right hip is bent and in an inward rotation, rather than an adduction.

▷ *Tip: With each inhalation, bring a little more length to your spine. Use this opportunity to twist a little further with each exhalation, and gently pull your right knee a little more to the left.*

But why are twists so good for back pain?

Rotational exercises like the Knee-down Twist and the Sitting Half Spinal Twist are simply good for our spines. They mobilise the thoracic spine and align the spine as a whole. The thoracic spine is one of the most mobile parts of the spine – or at least it should be. Unfortunately, this flexibility is gradually lost as a result of a lack of mobility or because of unequal tension. The lumbar spine, which is simply not designed for a large range of motion, compensates for this lack of mobility in the thoracic spine, and then becomes overexerted.

With twists, we bring movement back into the thoracic spine, so that the lumbar spine can once again focus on its role as a stabiliser.

Shoelace

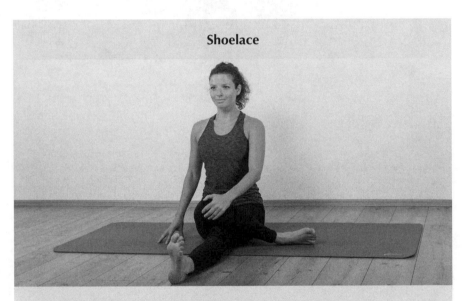

- Sit upright with your legs stretched out in front of you. Bend your right leg and lay it over the left leg. The outer edge or top of the right foot touches the floor near the left buttock.
- Bend the left leg and move the left heel closer to the right buttock. Manoeuvre the knees one on top of the other, as far as is comfortable for you.
- Bring your upper body into a slight forward bend. Surrender your leg and hip muscles to gravity.

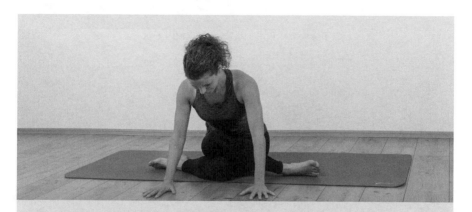

▷ **Tip:** *This pose is very demanding on the hips. Raise your sitting position with a thick cushion, so that the exercise is as comfortable as possible for your knees and spine.*

Baby Cradle

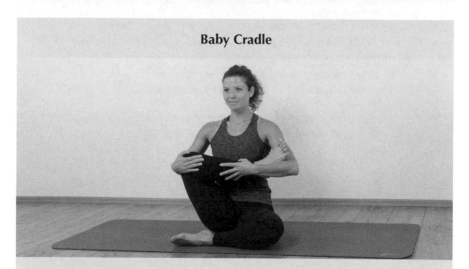

- Sit in a comfortable, upright position. Bend your right leg and pull it in to your upper body, twisting your knee outwards so that your right leg rotates outwards. Your knee should lie in your elbow crease. Hold your foot with your left hand.
- Gently rock your leg back and forth. This moves your thigh at the hip.
- You can control the intensity with your hands and arms. The closer you pull your lower leg, the more intense the stretch will feel.

▷ **Please note:** *Only move your thigh at the hip. Do not pull on your foot forcefully, as this places significant shear force on your knee.*

Forward Fold with Stacked Legs

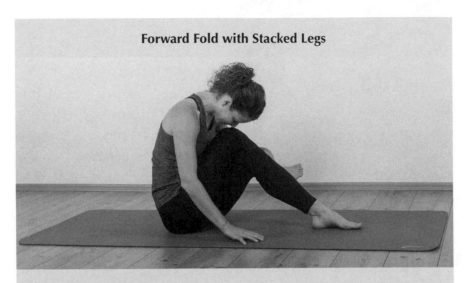

- Sit upright and stretch both legs out in front of you.
- Place your right foot above your left leg at knee height. Hold your right knee with your left hand and pull it as far as possible to the left.
- Lean your upper body forwards over your legs. Place your hands to the sides and let your upper body sink further forwards, without tension.

▷ **Tip:** *Be aware of your breathing. As you exhale, let go internally. Imagine all tension leaving your body as you exhale. You will feel that you can fold even further forwards.*

Seated Hurdle

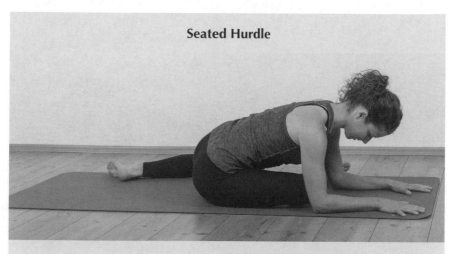

- Assume a tabletop starting position. Place your hands directly under your shoulders and your knees under your hips.
- Move the right leg forwards and the other to the side. Align your hips forwards – in other words, both hip bones face forwards.
- The right knee is at a right angle and points forwards. Slide the left leg to your left. The left knee is also at a 90-degree angle and lies on the floor.
- Lean your upper body forwards over your right leg. Support yourself on your forearms. Give your body a little time to soften.

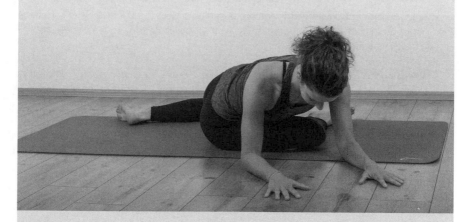

▷ **Tip:** *Move your upper body a little further to the right.*

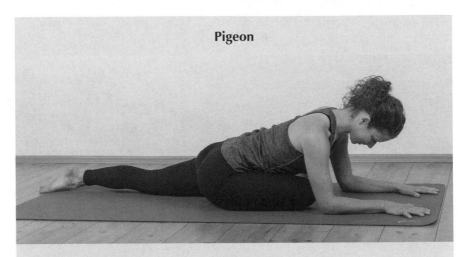

Pigeon

Pigeon is probably one of the most common exercises for the piriformis – and for good reason! In this passive, relatively relaxed posture, the hips are bent as much as possible and the stretch is most intense in the buttocks.

- Assume a tabletop position. Move your right knee forwards to your right hand. Stretch your left leg back as far as possible. The left groin expands and sinks down. The entire front of the left leg lies on the mat.
- Place your right lower leg diagonally in front of you on the mat, so that your right knee is behind your right elbow and your right foot is next to your left hip bone.
- Lay your upper body forwards onto your forearms. Give your body time to soften. After around 30 seconds, you can lay your upper body down completely and stretch your arms out forwards.

▷ **Please note:** *Exercise caution if you have knee problems! The bigger the angle in your front knee, the more intense the stretch in your buttocks; the smaller the angle, the weaker the stretch. However, be careful: if you apply a large angle but have little mobility in the hip, strong shear force can be exerted on the knee. Therefore, take it slow and easy.*

If you feel pressure in your back knee, you can move onto the toes of the back foot to reduce the pressure. Try it out!

Standing

You can do standing exercises anywhere, but we recommend practising near a wall, as all the exercises are carried out on one leg. This means that they are also good for stability training. Make sure that you focus on performing the stretch. For the first exercise, you will need a table for support.

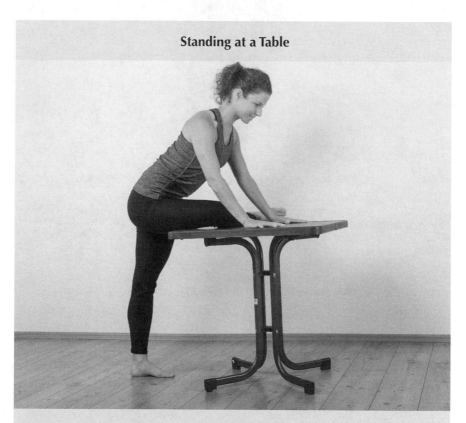

Standing at a Table

- Bend your leg and place it on the table, so that your outer thigh and outer lower leg are in contact with the table. The lower leg is parallel to the edge of the table. You will probably already feel a slight stretch in the buttocks.
- Lean forwards with your upper body. Move your hands as far forwards as possible and relax.

Half Chair Half Ankle to Knee Pose

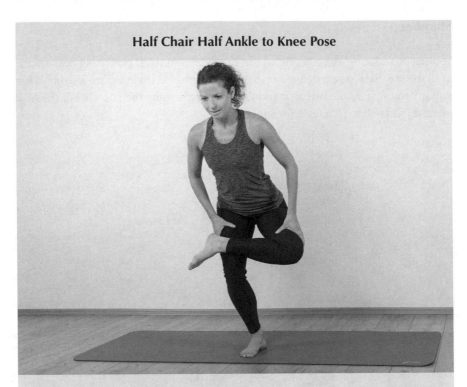

This is an exercise from yoga. As well as stretching the muscles in the buttocks and hips, it is particularly good for balance and stability. If you want to concentrate more fully on the stretching element, we recommend practising near a wall so that you can support yourself.

- Bend your left leg and rotate the knee outwards. Place the outside of your left foot on your right thigh just above your knee. The left thigh is already rotated outwards.
- Bend your knees. Move your buttocks backwards and tilt your upper body forwards so that your hips are more bent. The spine remains straight. The sternum lifts forwards.
- Place your left hand on your left thigh and gently rotate the thigh outwards and downwards. You should now be able to feel a stronger stretch in your buttocks. Keep the pressure gentle at first, otherwise too much stress is placed on the knees.

You can control the intensity with your standing leg and the upper body. The lower you go, the more you will feel the tension. The further you lean your upper body forwards, the more intense the stretch.

Revolved Triangle

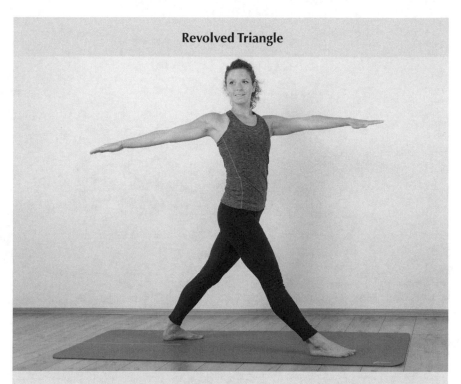

This is an advanced exercise that reaches not only the piriformis but also other hip muscles.

- Stand with your feet out wide, with the right leg forward. The right foot points forwards, and the left toes are at about 10 o'clock (in other words, turned outwards by 45 degrees).
- Actively straighten both legs. The thighs are engaged.
- Bring length into your spine and straighten your arms out to the sides. Keeping your spine long, turn your upper body to the right.

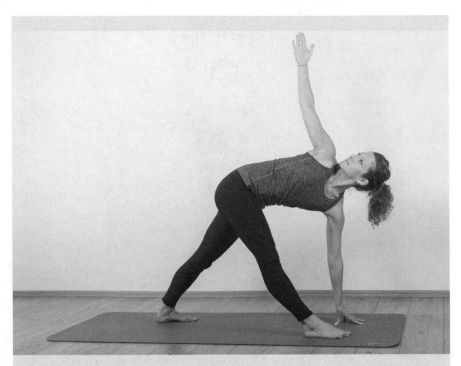

- Next lower your upper body towards the ground. The left hand touches the inside of your right foot. If this is too far away, place your left hand a little higher, on your leg or on a block or thick book.
- Now move your right buttock a little more upwards and outwards.

▷ **Tip:** *The more open your pelvis, the easier it is to keep your balance. Stagger your feet sideways a little for more stability.*

Make sure that both feet are fully in contact with the floor, which means that your adductors and internal rotators are obliged to work. They are the counterparts to the piriformis and the gluteus maximus. An imbalance between these two muscle groups can intensify piriformis syndrome.

Chair Exercises

Chairs are not just for sitting on! Exercises with a chair are perfect for relaxing the piriformis, even in the office.

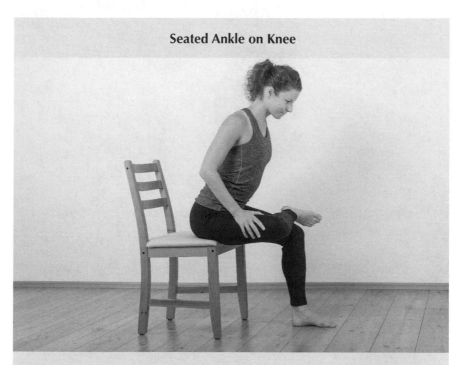

Seated Ankle on Knee

- Sit upright on the front edge of the chair, with both feet in contact with the floor.
- Place your right ankle on your left thigh, so that your right thigh is level in front of you.
- Bring your right hand to your right thigh, just above the knee, and your left hand to your left foot. Lengthen through your back and lean forwards.

You can control the intensity by increasing the pressure on your right thigh with your right hand. Do not go further than is comfortable for your knee.

Half Chair Half Ankle to Knee with Chair

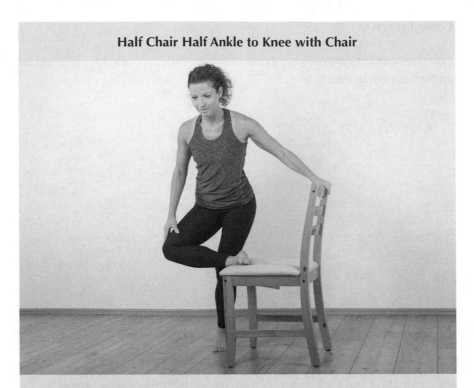

This exercise is similar to the standing version you encountered on p. 36, but is gentler on the knees, as your foot is lower because of the chair. This means that there is much less shear force acting on the knee.

- Stand with your left side in front of the chair. The seat of the chair points towards you.
- Hold the back of the chair with your left hand. Place the outer edge of your right foot on the seat of the chair. Relax your leg.
- Lengthen through your spine and lean forwards a little, gently bending your left leg (the supporting leg).

The further down you go, the more intense the stretch will be.

Stretches for Greater Mobility in the Hips

Limited mobility in the hips is a common issue that can be primarily attributed to our way of life. Sitting for hours on end, in combination with a lack of movement and loss of strength, has a negative effect on our physical condition. In addition, the hips are pivotal – in every sense of the word!

It is our hips and pelvis that connect the upper body to the lower body. Even minor imbalances, incorrect posture and issues relating to mobility and/or strength can bring the equilibrium between our upper and lower bodies or our left and right sides out of balance.

No muscle works completely alone – the piriformis is also dependent on the functioning of the other hip muscles. The following exercises will help you keep all your hip and pelvis muscles mobile.

Lumbar Area and Fronts of the Thighs: Function – Hip Flexors

Together with the thigh, sartorius, pectineus and tensor fasciae latae muscles, the large lumbar muscle – the psoas – and the iliacus muscle are responsible for moving the hips. These muscles are direct counterparts to the hip extensors, namely the muscles in the buttocks and the piriformis.

Sitting is a good example of hip flexor function. Regrettably, we generally sit much more than we should on a daily basis; moreover, our bodies are unfortunately excellent at adapting in this particular case. If we spend too much time in a position where our hips are bent, this then becomes their 'normal' position. Our bodies subsequently adapt: all the front structures become shortened, and the back ones become lengthened.

Anyone who spends a lot of time sitting should therefore stretch their hip flexors as well as the muscles in their buttocks in order to bring the pelvic alignment back into balance. To this end, the following exercises will help.

Lunge

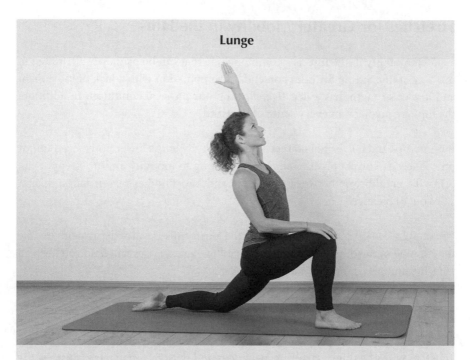

This exercise relaxes the hip flexors and thigh muscles and opens the entire front of the body. It is very satisfying to stretch the front of the body in this position, particularly if you have spent a long day sitting down.

- Assume a tabletop position. Now move your right foot forwards between your hands. Stretch your back leg as far backwards as you can, so that it is not lying directly on the kneecap.
- Let your left hipbone sink downwards. Give your hips a moment to soften.
- Support yourself with your right hand on your right thigh and align your upper body.

If you would like to go a little further, stretch your left arm upwards and imagine your sternum and hips pulling away from each other.

Thighs and Psoas with Chair

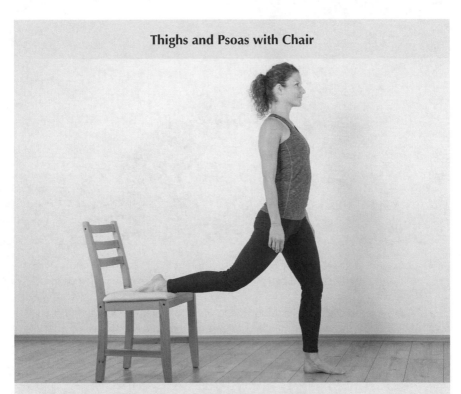

This is a very agreeable stretch that you can also practise easily in the office. If it is difficult for you to keep your balance on one leg, practise the exercise near a wall; this allows you to hold on at any time and concentrate on the stretch.

- Stand with your back to a chair. The distance between you and the chair should be between 50 cm and 1 m.
- Now place your right foot on the chair, so that only the top of your foot is in contact with the seat of the chair.
- Keep your upper body upright and your supporting leg straight. The knee of the leg on the chair points downwards at all times.
- Tilt your pelvis backwards slightly: to do this, pull your belly button in and move your hip bones forwards and up. Tilting your pelvis gives a greater stretch in the hip flexors and the fronts of your thighs.

▷ **Tip:** *The further your supporting leg is from the chair, the more you will reach the hip flexor muscles, since the hips are stretched more. If you stand closer to the chair, there is less stretching of the hips, which means the stretch is more intense in the thigh.*

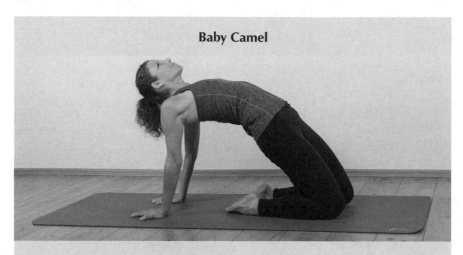

Baby Camel

- Come into a kneeling position, with your thighs parallel to each other. Place your hands on the ground behind your buttocks and turn your fingertips to face backwards.
- Slide your shoulders back and down and push your sternum forwards. Lift your buttocks from your heels. The hip bones move up towards the ceiling and the knees press down into the mat. Make sure to keep your knees together.
- Your head can hang backwards and relax. If this is uncomfortable for you, pull your chin towards your chest and look up to the ceiling.

Psoas and piriformis – a dream team

Thanks to their location, the psoas and piriformis are the only two muscles in our body that connect the legs and the spine. They are responsible for the alignment of the pelvis. In a healthy, even balance of forces, they work together efficiently, with the psoas pulling from the front and the piriformis from the back; unfortunately, however, this relationship can become imbalanced.

The Hamstrings: Function – Leg Flexors

Tension in the hamstrings brings the pelvis out of balance, so that it cannot be fully aligned. If you sit a lot, or often wear high heels for long periods, the backs of the legs tend to shorten.

The following exercises are very effective at reaching the backs of the legs. *Important*: when coming into a forward fold, keep your knees straight and move your upper body and hips.

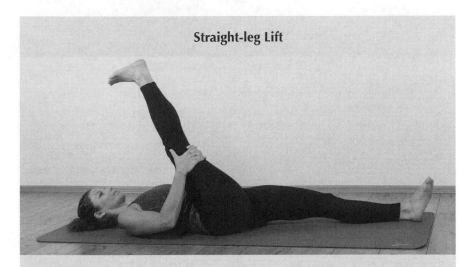

Straight-leg Lift

- Begin by lying on your back, and straighten your left leg out on the mat.
- Bend the right leg. Hold under your knee with your hands and pull your leg towards your upper body. You may like to stay here for a moment. You might already feel a pleasant stretch in the buttocks and lower back.
- Hold the back of your thigh with your hands and straighten the leg upwards. Actively push your heel upwards and pull the toes towards your nose. Press the right buttock into the mat in order to tense the whole back of the leg.
- The pelvis remains flat on the mat and both sides of the body are long. The left leg remains straight on the mat.

▷ **Tip:** *Use a hand towel or belt to help if you find it difficult to relax your upper body and your arms seem too short to hold your leg. Place the towel or belt around the back of your leg and hold both ends; this enables you to control the stretch yourself.*

Forward Fold

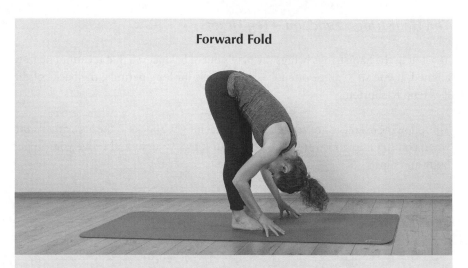

- Place your feet hip-width apart at most, and point your toes forwards so that your feet are parallel.
- Let your upper body sink down into a forward fold until your hands touch the floor. Bend your knees so that your fingertips reach the floor.
- Let your whole upper body hang and relax. Press your heels down into the floor, slide your sit bones upwards, and straighten your legs as much as you can; this stretches the entire backs of the legs.

Sitting Variation

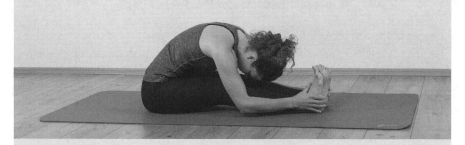

- Sit upright with your legs out straight in front of you.
- Lean forwards with your upper body. The hands are placed on the outsides of the legs, or you may be able to reach your ankles or toes.
- Let gravity pull you further and further down. Make sure to press the hollows of your knees down into the mat and point your toes upwards.

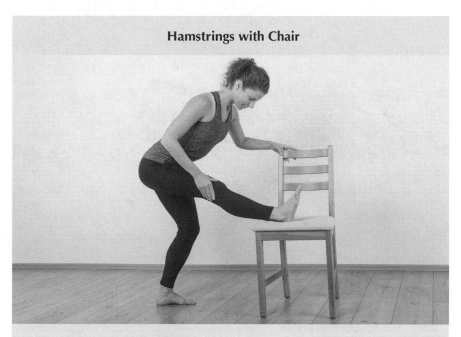

Hamstrings with Chair

- Stand in front of the chair. Place your right heel on the chair seat, with the toes pointing upwards. If you fully straighten your leg, you will probably feel a slight to moderate stretch in the back of your leg.
- Bend your standing leg a little and lean your upper body forwards from your hips.
- Actively push your left buttock back a little, so that both hip bones are aligned.

The Inner Thighs: Function – Raising the Leg

The muscles in the inner thigh are also called the *adductors*, and include five different muscles; their main role is to pull the thigh up to the core of the body. When you walk, these muscles stabilise the leg axes and pelvis, thus taking on an important role with regard to the stability of the pelvis and knee. If they are overexerted or tense, they tend to be inflamed or have structural injuries, such as tears and strains. With the following exercises, you can prevent this and keep your hips mobile.

Lying Butterfly

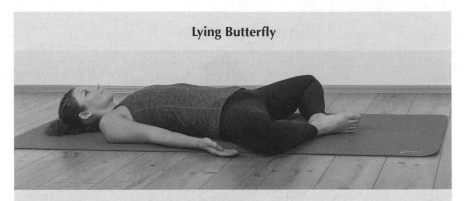

- Lie on your back and place your feet near your buttocks. Let your knees fall out to the sides and bring the soles of your feet together.
- The knees naturally move downwards.
- Close your eyes and inhale deeply, before exhaling even more deeply. As you exhale, release any tension from your hips. You will feel your hips gradually opening – simply as a result of your breathing and gravity.
- Let your whole body relax.

Hips and emotions – the psycho-emotional level

Stretching the adductors provides relief to our hips. Anyone who sits a lot will find it very satisfying to open and expand the hips using adductor stretches. Hip-opening exercises, however, are also good for us on an emotional level – they relax us. Why is that? Our hips are like a hidden 'physical memory'.

Emotions such as fear and sadness, as well as stress and traumatic events, are stored in the hips – hidden perhaps, but still present. Often, hip pain occurs in moments of emotional stress. Relaxing the hip muscles, particularly the inner thighs and psoas (see p. 44), is important not just for our physical well-being, but for our emotional well-being too.

Standing Angle

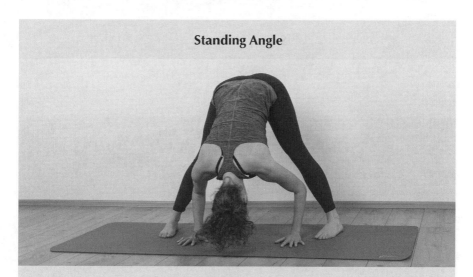

Standing or sitting in straddle positions stretches both the inner thighs and the backs of the legs (see p. 45). If you press your heels down into the floor, and at the same time push your sit bones up towards the ceiling, you will feel the stretch just as strongly in the backs of your legs as in your inner thighs.

- Take a wide stance – your feet should be wider than hip-width apart. Point your toes forwards and straighten your legs.
- Place your hands on your hips and sink your upper body down, keeping length in the spine. When you have come down as far as possible, release your hands from your hips and place them on the floor/mat.
- Let your upper body hang down, and relax.

▷ **Please note:** *Move slowly into the final position and avoid forcing yourself deeper into the stretch. This applies to all stretches, but in this one you should be particularly careful, as the inner thighs are very sensitive.*

Sitting Variation

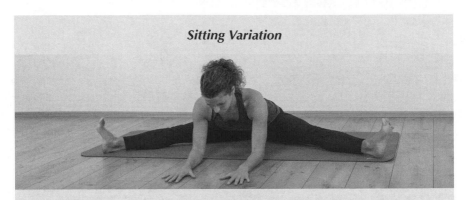

- Sit on a mat with your legs apart. The further away from each other you place your legs, the more intense the stretch will be.
- Move your upper body forwards as far as comfortably possible. Make sure that your little toes point outwards, as this causes your thighs to rotate inwards.

Inner Thighs with Chair

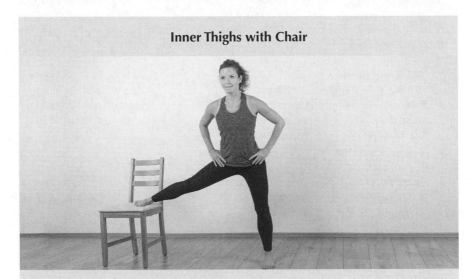

- Stand with your side to a chair and place the inside of the foot closest to the chair on the seat.
- The leg on the chair remains completely straight.
- Make sure that both hip bones are facing forwards. The toes of the foot on the chair face forwards and the heel is pressed away from you.
- Bend your standing leg a little to increase the stretch in the inner thigh of the leg on the chair.

7

Myofascial Relaxation

What is Fascia?

Fascia is currently a hot topic – and for good reason. No other tissue has garnered such attention and interest in a long time. But why is this?

In principle, fascia is simply connective tissue. Thanks to new scientific methods, we now know that not only does it play a connective role, but also it is very active tissue with many functions in the body, including stability and the transfer of forces.

Healthy fascia is elastic. However, under- and overexertion, incorrect stresses and injuries can change the tissue, limiting its suppleness. Fascia tends to 'stick' if it is not used, or used more on one side of the body. This stickiness first takes the form of tension that you can usually feel with your hands. Since everything in our bodies is connected, these tensions then affect our stability and the quality of our movements.

But what has this got to do with the piriformis? Well, piriformis pain is often a tension problem. You can target the affected area yourself with a ball or fascia roller.

> **Fascia and back pain**
>
> Scientists have proved that in patients with chronic back pain, the lumbar fascia (the largest back fascia, situated in the lower back) is much firmer and thicker than in those with no pain. Furthermore, studies have shown that there are many pain receptors in the back fascia; this means that when dealing with back pain, it is important to take the muscles and fascia into consideration, and not just the intervertebral discs.

Rolling – What Is It and What Happens?

Rolling connective tissue has a similar effect to massage. The aim is to press old, exhausted connective tissue fluids out of the fascia, because they gradually fill up with metabolic waste products. After this has been done, fresh fluids can then impregnate the tissue. You can visualise this process as a sponge from which you are wringing out toxins and lymphatic fluids. The sponge then fills up again with new fluids – this means the fascia network remains properly hydrated and supple. You can also massage painful tense and sticky areas with rollers and balls.

What Do You Need?

A fascia roller is sufficient. If you also use a ball (even a tennis ball), you can actively target both large and small painful areas. A wide range of rollers and balls are now available on the market, with various lengths, degrees of hardness and structures. We recommend a softer roller, even for acute issues, so that you can really work slowly and with awareness, without further stimulating the pain receptors.

Effective Rolling

Rolling speed – the essentials
We recommend rolling very slowly. Use your breathing as a guide. One centimetre per breath is a good reference.

Painful areas – the trigger point

Even if you work selectively with the ball, you will undoubtedly find areas that are particularly painful or stuck. This is particularly true for the piriformis. Roll especially slowly and with awareness in this case.

Intensity – less is more

The fascia is densely populated with pain receptors; it is therefore essential not to overdo it! Do not go beyond your pain threshold.

Duration – give yourself time

Because you are rolling slowly, each part will take two to three minutes. Leave enough time to massage both sides. Contrary to intensity, where 'too much' should be avoided, you can certainly be a little more ambitious when it comes to duration – up to five minutes is acceptable.

Reaching the area

Piriformis massage is actually not so easy, as the piriformis is somewhat hidden under the gluteus maximus and is hard to feel. You can best reach the area with a fascia ball, or a tennis or lacrosse ball, as these have a smaller surface area than a roller, meaning that you can work stuck tissue in a more targeted way.

The roller works better on larger surfaces. The effect described above, whereby the tissue is pressed to rehydrate it, can be better achieved in this way. This is why combining the roller and the ball is the most sensible choice – include both variations in your training!

We recommend that you also include the other structures around the hip (the iliotibial band and the thigh) in your rolling.

Rolling the Piriformis with a Ball

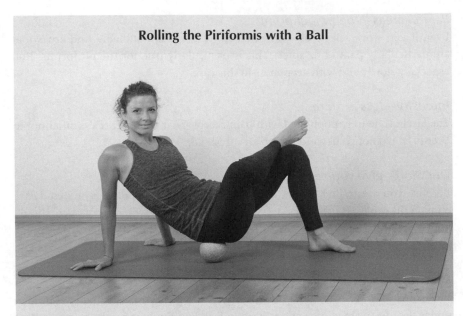

- Place the ball under the right buttock, so that you can roll the side area with the ball and are not sitting on it with your sit bones.
- Support yourself with your hands on the floor behind you. Pay attention to your shoulders! Move your sternum upwards and your shoulders down.
- Roll the gluteus maximus and the entire side of the buttock with small, circular movements. You will find that some areas are relatively relaxed and others more painful. Stay in the latter areas for a moment. You will probably identify the piriformis very quickly.
- Roll slowly with the ball, as the piriformis is somewhat hidden. If you roll over the piriformis quickly, you will not go deep enough into the tissue to reach it.

Rolling the Piriformis with a Roller

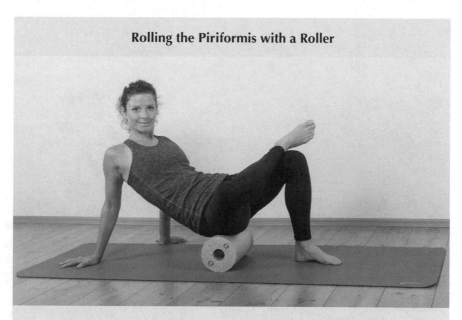

- Sit on the roller, with your feet on the floor. Support yourself with your hands on the floor behind you. Pay attention to your shoulders! Move your sternum upwards and your shoulders down.
- Place your right foot on your left thigh and transfer your weight to the right half of your buttocks.
- Roll slowly forwards and backwards from the sit bones to the sacral bone.
- Even if the piriformis is not targeted as directly with the roller as with the ball, you will be able to identify the area, especially if you struggle with acute tension in the piriformis.
- Gently stay in the stuck areas for a moment and breathe deeply three or four times with awareness. Then slowly continue rolling.

Outer Thighs – The Iliotibial Band

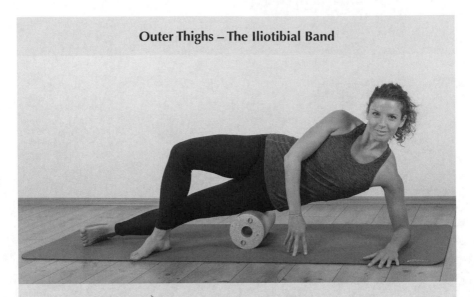

- Lie on your side, using your arm to support you, and place the roller under the outer thigh. Now straighten both legs.
- Move your top leg forwards. You can also place your upper hand in front of your body for support. Press up from your supporting shoulder.
- Roll the outer thigh slowly between the knee and the hip. Give yourself time and stay in any places that you feel need more work, or use small rolling movements to specifically address them.

▷ *Tip: If massage using the roller on the floor is too painful, you can use a ball (or tennis ball) against a wall. In this variation, roll the entire outer thigh using small, circular movements; this places much less weight on the area being rolled.*

Thighs

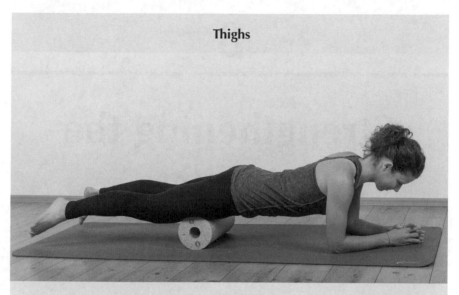

- Kneel on the mat and place the roller just in front of your knees.
- Support yourself on your forearms, so that the roller is now under your thighs. Activate your abdominal muscles and keep your shoulders stable. Your body is parallel to the floor.
- Now move your whole body forwards from your shoulder joint, rolling the thighs down to just above the knee – but no further. From here, move back from your shoulders and roll in the other direction.

▷ **Tip:** *Vary the rolling movements: while rolling, turn your toes inwards and outwards in order to reach the inner and outer parts of the large thigh muscles.*

8

Strengthening the Muscles

What Strength Training Can Do for You

In addition to the aesthetic aspects, regular strength training has many positive effects on health:

- Higher bone density, stronger muscles and stronger connective tissue
- Lower risk of injury
- Greater muscle mass and higher basal metabolic rate
- Better quality of life
- Reduction in muscular imbalances

It is also sensible to strengthen the muscles if you have sciatica or piriformis syndrome. In principle, regular strength training in combination with mobility training is the best preventive measure you can take in order to remain free of complaints.

In acute cases, it is also sensible to carry out the exercises to release tension (from p. 23); they will rapidly have a positive effect and can relieve pain. However, in the long term it is important to deal with the cause of the problem, and strength training is the first step to doing this.

In the following section, we have put together a selection of exercises for which you do not need anything apart from your own body and a mat. For exercise progression, in other words for increasing the intensity, the mini-band is used, which is a super training tool for outer rotation and abduction.

Recommendations for Strength Training

We have collected three outer rotation, three abduction and three buttock-activating exercises for you, plus a combination exercise that brings together outer rotation and abduction. As a minimal session, you can take *one exercise from each section* and add the *combination exercise*. Of course, you can also select more exercises if you wish.

You should complete the exercises *two to three times per week*. It is best to have a rest day in between in order to regenerate.

The number of repetitions varies depending on the exercise and the training level. Some exercises are calculated in terms of duration rather than number of repetitions. We therefore give *individual recommendations for each exercise;* most suggest between *10 and 15 repetitions*.

We recommend that the set of exercises is repeated *two or three times*.

You should always practise the exercises in a *slow and controlled* manner.

Outer Rotation

The piriformis is a strong outer rotator when the hips are straight. Exercises that rotate the thigh outwards in the hip can target the muscle in the most effective way.

Standing Toes Outwards

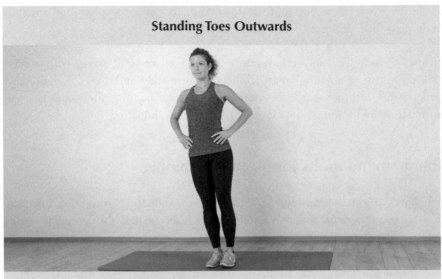

- Stand upright. Bring length to your whole body.
- Transfer your weight to your right foot and gently lift your left foot from the floor. The toes point forwards.
- Rotate your whole left leg outwards. The movement comes from the hip, and the leg remains straight. At the end of the movement, your toes point to the left, or front left, depending on your degree of mobility. Your knee also points to the left.

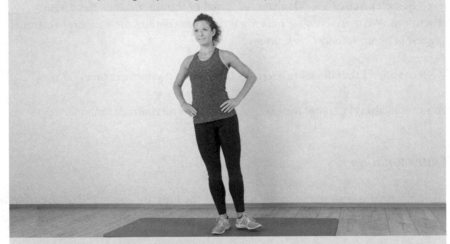

Recommendation: 12 to 15 repetitions per side.

Practise this exercise close to a wall for support if you wobble. The outer rotation of the hip is more important than standing steadily on one leg.

Tree

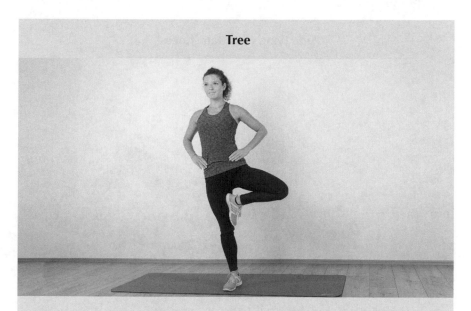

- Stand upright. Anchor your feet to the mat and point your toes forwards.
- Transfer your weight to your right leg and lift your left foot from the floor. Hold your left knee with both hands and pull it towards your body. The upper body remains upright, and the standing leg is strong and sturdy.
- Now turn the left leg out from the hip joint and place the left foot on the inside of the right thigh.
- Actively press the sole of the foot and the thigh against each other.
- Point your left knee outwards, without twisting the hip. Both hip bones continue to point forwards, while the left leg is in an outer rotation.

Recommendation: Hold for 10 breaths (45 to 60 seconds) per side.

If you are not able to place your foot on your inner thigh, simply place it a little lower on your inner lower leg. If you have difficulty balancing, you can place the tip of your foot on the floor and turn the knee outwards. The main thing is that the knee points outwards, so that you maintain the outer rotation.

Stay focused. Find a fixed point on which to focus all your attention – that way you will be much more stable.

Side Lying with Bent Knees

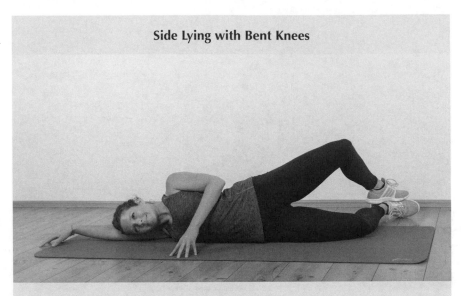

- Lie on your side. Bend your knees at a 90-degree angle, so that your feet lie behind you. The hips remain straight. You can lay your upper body on your lower arm and allow it to relax. Stabilise yourself to the side with your upper arm.
- Lift the knee of your top leg upwards. The feet remain closed; the inner arches of the feet touch throughout the exercise.
- Lower the knee again and then repeat the lifting of the knee.

Recommendation: 10 to 12 repetitions per side.

In order to address the function of the piriformis as a strong outer rotator, it is essential to keep the feet together throughout the whole exercise. Another detail not to be forgotten is the straight hips. The piriformis is strongest as an outer rotator when the hips are straight.

▷ **Tip:** *With the use of a mini-band (see p. 66), you can increase the resistance in order to achieve a higher level of strength. For this exercise, the mini-band is placed on the thigh, just above the knee. Start with 10 repetitions per side.*

Abduction

Abduction is the action of splaying the legs outwards (away from the centre of the body). The piriformis is not a traditional abductor, but it does support the muscles responsible for abduction.

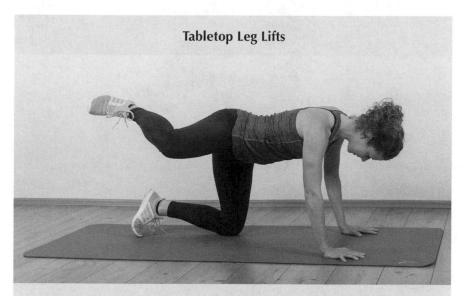

Tabletop Leg Lifts

- Assume a tabletop position. Place your hands directly under your shoulders and your knees under your hips. Anchor your hands firmly to the mat so that your shoulders remain stable. Bring length to your spine. The head is an extension of the cervical spine.
- Lift your right leg to the side. The knee stays at a right angle. Bring the leg up as far as your mobility allows.
- At the highest point, the toes point outwards. Both shoulders are in alignment and the pelvis remains in its neutral position.

Recommendation: 12 repetitions per side.

Seated Press

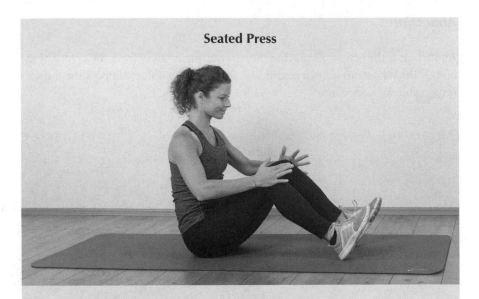

The Seated Press is an isometric exercise.

- Sit with your feet flat on the floor. Your knees are hip-width apart.
- Place your palms on your outer thighs, just above the knees. Press inwards with your palms. Press against your hands with your legs, so that your knees stay hip-width apart.
- Your legs work outwards. Apply constant pressure outwards.

Recommendation: Carry out the exercise for 45 seconds, quickly releasing the tension from time to time.

Pay attention to your breathing. The consistent build-up of pressure can often lead to you holding your breath. Continue to breathe normally and take short breaks.

Isometric training

The word *isometric* is a compound of *iso-*, meaning 'equal', and *metric*, meaning 'relating to measurement'. In isometric exercises, the muscle length does not change on contraction; in other words, there is no movement of the joint. Only static strain is used – the muscles are activated using pushing or pulling exercises, but remain static.

Of course, strength training should not include just isometric exercises; such exercises, however, are perfect as short breaks and for directly targeting individual muscle groups.

Standing One-leg Lift

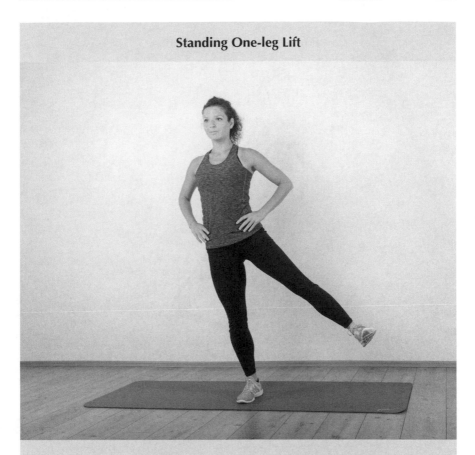

- Stand upright and transfer your weight to your right leg. Bend your right leg slightly. Point your left toes outwards, so that the majority of your weight is now on your standing leg (the right).
- Lift the tip of your left foot from the floor. Push your heel away from you. Lift your left leg up as far as the strength and mobility in your hip allow.
- At the highest point, the toes point forwards. The heel is the furthest point away from you. The hips remain aligned and neutral; in other words, the hips are approximately level. Your posture remains upright.
- Slowly lower your leg again in a controlled manner until just above the floor, before lifting it again.

Recommendation: 15 repetitions per side.

Progression with Mini-band

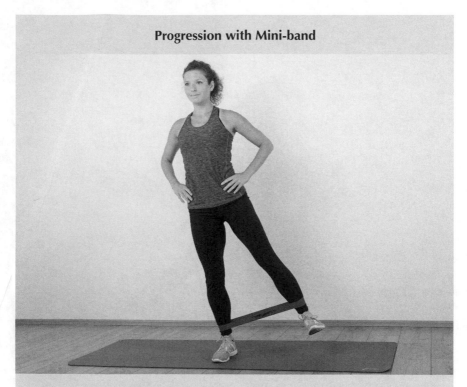

If you would like to increase the resistance when splaying your legs, the mini-band is a good option.

- Place the band above the ankles. Ensure that it lies flat and is not twisted.
- The exercise is then carried out as described in the 'Standing One-leg Lift', page 65. Splay the legs and stretch the mini-band. In addition to gravity and bodyweight, resistance against the band now comes into play.

Recommendation: 10 to 12 repetitions per side.

The mini-band – a small but effective training tool

The mini-band is a wide circular elastic band, available in various strengths. As it is small, light and cheap, it is a wonderful training tool for at home and when away. You can use it to easily increase the resistance (and thus the difficulty) of many exercises.

The mini-band has migrated from the therapy and competitive sports domains to the health and fitness sector.

Combination Exercise – Outer Rotation with Abduction

The following exercise combines outer rotation and abduction and is thus particularly demanding and effective.

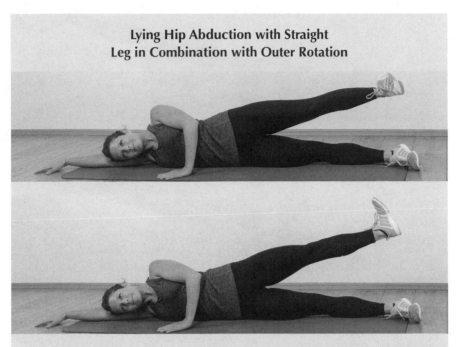

Lying Hip Abduction with Straight Leg in Combination with Outer Rotation

- Lie on your side so that your body forms a straight line and the pelvis is stacked vertically.
- You can relax your head onto your bottom arm, and support yourself by placing the top arm in front of you. Bring tension to your whole body.
- Lift your top leg, keeping it straight, to around 45 degrees. Push your heel away from you. The toes point forwards. This movement is called *abduction* – your leg moves away from your body.

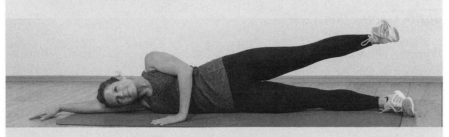

- Now turn your leg outwards, so that your toes point almost vertically upwards. Your leg remains completely straight. This provides the external rotation.

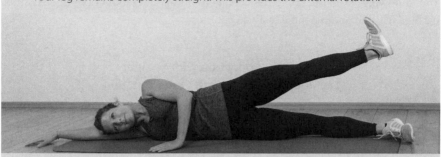

- Next, turn your leg inwards again in order to return to the abduction position.

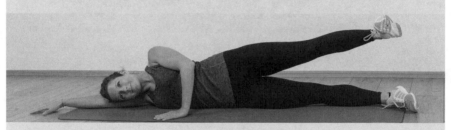

- Lower the leg.
- Lift – rotate outwards – return to abduction position – lower. Repeat this sequence several times, taking care to perform each position properly.

Recommendation: 10 to 12 repetitions per side

Throughout the whole exercise, make sure that your pelvis remains stacked vertically and does not lean forwards or backwards.

Buttock Activation

With the following exercises, we specifically target the muscles in the buttocks. There are several muscles in this region:

- Large buttock muscle (gluteus maximus)
- Medium buttock muscle (gluteus medius)
- Small buttock muscle (gluteus minimus).

These muscles all work together with the hip muscles, including the piriformis (see the 'Piriformis Syndrome and Athletes' chapter, p. 78).

The gluteus maximus is the largest and one of the strongest muscles in our bodies. However, because of our increasingly inactive lifestyles, particularly with the amount of time we spend sitting down, our buttock muscles are continually becoming weaker. The less we actively use a muscle, the greater the danger that our body will forget to use it. The nervous system plays an important role here.

The following exercises should help to keep your buttock muscles healthy in their partnership with the hip muscles.

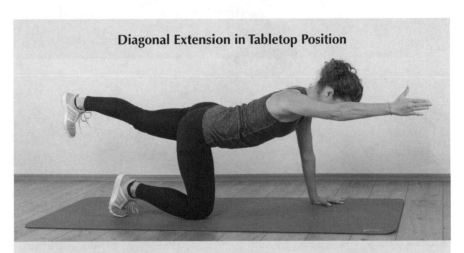

Diagonal Extension in Tabletop Position

- Assume a tabletop position. Place your hands directly under your shoulders and your knees under your hips. Anchor your hands to the mat, so that your shoulders remain stable. Bring length to your spine. The head is an extension of the cervical spine.
- At the same time straighten your right arm forwards and your left leg backwards, so that your arm, upper body and leg form a line parallel to the floor. Create length in your body. Push the fingertips forwards and the toes backwards, away from each other. This tension brings stability to the pose.
- Using small movements, lift and lower the back leg a little. The toes always point downwards.

Recommendation: Hold the position for 30 seconds on each side, or lift the leg slightly 15 times.

Dynamic variation

Lift your right arm and left leg, then return them to the floor straight away. Change onto the other side immediately, and lift your left arm and right leg. Return to the floor and change to the other side. If you like, you can synchronise the movements with your breathing: as you inhale, lift your arm and leg, then lower them as you exhale.

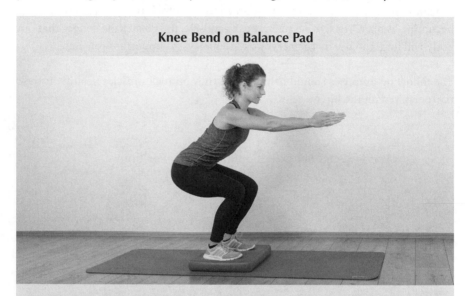

Knee Bend on Balance Pad

The knee bend is performed on an unstable surface, with the aim of encouraging the interaction between nerves and muscles. Of course, you can also do this exercise on a stable surface – activation of the buttock muscles will still take place.

- Stand upright with the feet shoulder-width apart. The toes point forwards.
- Now move your buttocks down and back until your thighs are parallel with the floor. The knees are in line with or behind the toes in order to reduce strain on the knee joints. Keeping the spine straight, gently lean the upper body forwards and stretch your arms out in front of you.
- Return to an upright position. As you come back up, activate your buttock muscles with awareness. Do not fully straighten your knees. Then sink down again.

Recommendation: 15 repetitions.

▷ **Tip:** *You can also work with the mini-band for this exercise in order to reach the gluteus maximus in addition to the abductors and the lateral buttock muscles. In this case, place the mini-band on the thigh just above the knee.*

Bridge with Mini-band

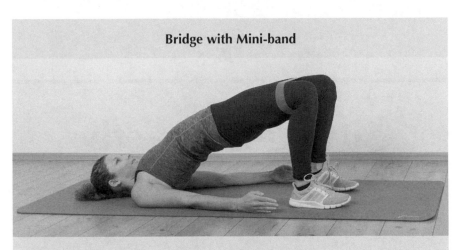

For this exercise, the mini-band is used as an additional tool. When placed on the thighs, the band adds resistance for training the abduction force (i.e. the splaying of the legs). Of course, you can also do this exercise without the mini-band.

- Lie on your back. Place your feet hip-width apart, near your buttocks. Your knees are also hip-width apart.
- Position the mini-band around the middle of your thighs. Relax your upper body. The arms rest at the sides of the body.
- Lift your pelvis up until your shoulders, pelvis and knees are in a diagonal line at the highest point.
- Now activate your buttock muscles and push your hip bones further upwards.

9

Sitting Correctly

Sitting a lot, and incorrectly, is one of the most common causes of back pain. This also applies to piriformis syndrome – sitting tensely for long periods is one of its main causes.

Modern Lifestyles

In our everyday lives, most activities are performed sitting down. In the morning, we sit in the car or on the train to get to work. We work sitting at a desk. At lunch, we sit to eat, then return to our desks. After work, it is back to the car or the train. And when you finally get home after a hard day at work, you cannot wait for a good meal and a few hours on the sofa – which, of course, involves plenty of sitting!

As you can see, we spend much of our lives sitting, although our bodies are absolutely not intended for this. They are designed for the lifestyle of our ancestors – hard physical labour and many miles on foot. The best solution, of course, would be to transform our posture patterns, but unfortunately in most cases this is not possible. We therefore need to make sure that we are at least sitting properly!

Masters of sitting

On average, adults in industrialised countries sit for 50 to 60% of the day; in other words, of the 15 to 18 hours we are awake, we spend 8 to 12 hours sitting. How many hours a day do you spend sitting? Keep a 'sitting journal' for two or three days. You will be surprised – and perhaps a little shocked – at how many hours you spend sitting down.

The Piriformis Suffers

When we sit, we place constant pressure on the piriformis; this results in a metabolic deficit in the muscles, leading to cramps and shortened muscles in this area. Remember that when you sit for long periods, the muscle is permanently contracted. Over time, this leads to pathological changes (tension).

Moreover, the piriformis is not the only muscle affected by too much sitting. The muscles in the backs of the thighs, namely the hamstrings (biceps femoris, semimembranosus and semitendinosus), tend to become shortened, although this is reversible. The hip flexor muscles and abdominal muscles become weakened, leading to an unnatural alignment of the spine, not only when you sit, but also over the long term when you stand and walk.

Be careful not to sit on your money!

Many people (especially men) carry their wallets in their back trouser pockets. When standing and walking this is not a problem, but if you constantly sit on your wallet, this increases the inflammation and compression of the piriformis.

Correct Sitting Technique

In principle, you should make sure to change your sitting position as often as possible: three to four times per hour would be good, as this means the body is constantly adjusting to new stresses. Slumping back into your chair is therefore permitted – as long as you sit upright in between periods of slumping.

To optimise the design of your workplace, we recommend taking the following points into account:

- The seat of your chair should be at approximately the height of the hollows of your knees. Your upper and lower legs should form at least a 90-degree angle, or preferably even larger: 100 to 110 degrees. You can better align your pelvis on a slightly downward-sloping seat.
- Use the whole seat and the backrest. Sit upright, so that at least two thirds of your thighs are on the seat.
- The desk is at the perfect height if your keyboard is at elbow level. Set up your monitor, so that the upper edge of the screen is at about eye level, and you can look directly at your screen.

Essentially, it is recommended that the pelvis should be aligned when you are sitting – in other words, avoiding a rounded back. However, as already mentioned, it can be a good idea to slouch and relax from time to time.

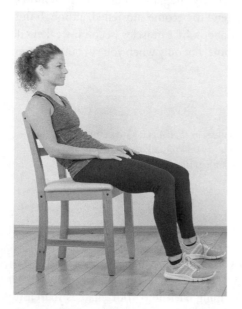 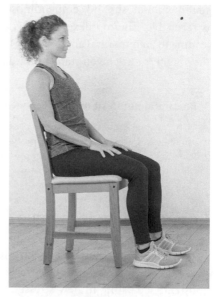

The pelvis is tilted backwards, causing unnatural pressure on the intervertebral discs in the lumbar spine area. The thoracic spine is curved more than usual.

The pelvis is upright, and the spine is aligned in its natural S curve, so that forces are optimally distributed.

10

Additional Measures

Treating piriformis syndrome requires a lot of patience and perseverance: it can take several weeks, or even months, until the symptoms completely disappear. This book follows a movement-oriented approach to treatment, but recovery can be supported by various other measures.

Pain-relief and Anti-inflammatory Medications

In acute cases, as a first step doctors often prescribe pain-relief and anti-inflammatory medications, such as diclofenac, ibuprofen and coxibs. These NSAIDs (nonsteroidal anti-inflammatory drugs) are readily available and quickly reduce pain. However, caution should be exercised with regard to their long-term use, not only because of side effects but also on account of the fact that these medications do not deal with the underlying issues, and therefore do not provide a long-term solution to the problem. Nevertheless, medication can provide short-term relief.

Acupuncture

Acupuncture is an element of traditional Chinese medicine (TCM). In this context, the body is thought to contain a life-force energy and to be full of pathways that distribute this energy throughout our bodies. On these pathways, there are many acupuncture points that are locally stimulated to release blockages.

Acupuncture can support the healing process and the search for the causes of piriformis syndrome.

Osteopathy

Osteopathy is an alternative branch of medicine; the body is regarded as a functional unit, which is basically responsible for autoregulation.

Osteopaths primarily work with the connective tissues (fascia), which link together everything within the body. By using a special fascial technique, connective tissue massage can detect and release tensions in the musculofascial system.

Ultrasound

Ultrasound therapy is an alternative therapy procedure. For this, short consecutive ultrasound waves are transferred directly to the body, which has the effect of making the tissue relax.

Heat or Cold

Heat can be very beneficial for releasing the hardened structures in tense muscles. Saunas, baths and heat cushions are particularly suitable for this.

Cold should be used if nerves are inflamed. It should first be determined whether the pain is due to tense muscles or to nerve inflammation.

Kinesiology Taping

Even in acute cases, treatment with tape can quickly provide relief from pain. The tape used is mobile, elastic and breathable. Unlike in traditional taping, which is designed to limit movement, kinesiology taping works using the physiology of the skin.

The tape sticks to the top layer of the skin, so that the blood can circulate better in the injured areas; this improves the reaction of blood vessels and nerves. Furthermore, the tissue under the kinesiology tape will be better supplied with oxygen. Waste products in the tissue, as well as substances that can cause muscle fatigue, are removed more quickly. In this way, kinesiology taping ensures better regeneration, or recovery, of the tissue.

11

Piriformis Syndrome and Athletes

Those who lead sedentary lives are not the only ones affected by piriformis syndrome. In addition to an under-exertion and incorrect use of muscles, an overuse or a mixture of various elements can also have painful consequences.

Piriformis syndrome frequently affects runners and triathletes. The piriformis is placed under excessive stress as a result of a poor running technique, high volumes of training and increasing training volumes too rapidly. Uneven surfaces and running in old shoes can also increase the stress on already burdened structures. Anyone who trains a lot for their sport often forgets to include general strength training as well as running, cycling or swimming.

When the primary muscles used get tired, the smaller auxiliary muscles, such as the piriformis, work harder to avoid inappropriate stresses. However, the limits of these smaller muscles are also reached at a certain point – and they consequently react with tension, irritation or even inflammation.

Do not increase your running distance too quickly

As a rule of thumb, do not increase your running by more than 10% per week – this applies to beginners and more ambitious athletes alike. The less time the body has for getting used to stresses, the more likely injuries become.

As a runner, you should pay attention to the following external risk factors:

- Running too far
- Increasing the running distance too quickly
- Poor running technique
- Worn shoes
- Running for long periods on uneven surfaces

If you can avoid as many of these external factors as possible, you may be able to prevent internal issues, such as poor posture and muscular imbalances, and may even strengthen the hip and pelvis muscles.

Studies have shown that greater hip strength significantly reduces running injuries. Particularly with knee problems, it makes sense to work on stabilising the hips in order to relieve pain. Furthermore, increasing the stride length, which goes hand in hand with increasing hip strength, can also lead to improved performance.

In the 'Strengthening the Muscles' chapter (p. 58), you can find exercises to strengthen the hip-stabilising muscles.

Iliotibial band syndrome (ITBS) – a common complaint among runners

Iliotibial band syndrome, often called *runner's knee*, makes itself felt in the form of increasing pain on the outside of the knee. In this case, strengthening the muscles in the torso and hips can help. As the cause of this painful condition is usually a weakening of the small muscles in the buttocks, it often results in imbalances between the left and right sides. In addition, it can be useful to roll the outer thigh with a fascia roller (see p. 56) and to stretch the area (see the 'Releasing Tension' chapter, p. 23).

12

Conscious Movement is the Best Prevention and Therapy

D r Torsten Pfitzer is an expert in the field of holistic pain management, with a practice in Munich. For him, a holistic approach to piriformis syndrome is essential. In this interview, he answers some key questions.

Are there specific sports that you recommend for those with piriformis syndrome?

A simple list of recommended sports would not be suitable for this complex subject. It is more a question of the diversity of the movement and the quality of the sport, for avoiding long-term issues.

Additional exercises are suitable for this condition, for every type of sport; these ensure an optimal balance of tension in the muscle-fascia network, which runs throughout the whole body. Certain forms of yoga, Pilates and Qi Gong are helpful, as they also place great importance on breathing. Of course, the exercises given in this book are well suited, as they specifically train the muscles and fascia in the pelvic area in terms of length and strength.

Which sports should be avoided?

Sports that require one-sided, monotonous movements generally carry a higher risk of inappropriate stresses and overexertion than those that incorporate a variety of movements. The kick used for swimming breaststroke is also not recommended if you already have problems with the piriformis.

There is no single sport, however, that has a significantly higher risk of causing piriformis syndrome. It's more helpful to ask yourself 'How do I practise this sport?' and 'What other circumstances favour the development of the condition?'

Here's a quick example: piriformis syndrome often occurs in runners and triathletes. The reason for this is the intensity of the sport they do, which commonly leads to overexertion, either as a result of the duration or an overly rapid increase in distances. Today, it is fairly common for leisure joggers, who spend most of their days sitting in an office, to have taken on a half-marathon, or at least participated in a company race. Many people, however, do not have a suitable balance of tension for such challenges. In other words, even when resting, there is too much tension in some areas of the muscle-fascia network, and not enough in others. The structures designed for stability and movement can then no longer keep up, and so the small piriformis muscle tries to take on their work and compensate. However, as this is not the function of the piriformis, the muscle becomes tense and stiff relatively quickly.

With jogging, to stay with a relatively common, popular sport, other factors, such as running style and shoes, can of course also lead to incorrect stresses. Thus, my recommendation is not to avoid certain sports as a preventive measure, but rather, as mentioned above, to notice one-sided tensions promptly and above all to practise more relaxed, balanced leisure sports – without the competitive element.

If you already have a stiff piriformis muscle, it is a good idea to gradually return to exercising during or after treatment, after consulting with your doctor or therapist.

Are buttock pain, back pain and shoulder pain connected?

Oh yes, absolutely! And it is incredibly important to take this into consideration in training and therapy. Today, we are very familiar with the development of myofascial chains; these are defined pathways of muscles and fascia that connect various parts of the skeleton in three dimensions, mostly from the head to the feet. Organ functions and their reliance on fascia often also play a role in functional muscular disorders, particularly if they occur on both sides of the body.

If you think of the body as an interactive unit, it quickly becomes clear that a problem in one area can continue in another area, and will do so over time. Our body is a master at compensating, in other words balancing out issues. This means that pain does not necessarily occur at the same place as the cause, but rather where there is most tension, for example if the latter can no longer be compensated for by further stresses.

From an osteopathic perspective, there are various patterns which, in the case of misalignment, continue across specific parallel areas, such as the skull, the shoulders and the pelvic area, and further afield to the knees and ankles. So, for example, misalignments at the base of the skull can cause the spine, shoulders, back and pelvis/buttocks to twist. On the other hand, a rotation between the pelvis and sacral bone (sometimes referred to as the sacroiliac joint) can, over time, wear out certain ligaments, causing the piriformis muscle to attempt to maintain stability in the pelvic area by tensing up. As this stabilising function is not one of its intended roles, it quickly cramps, and this (either alone or often by compressing the sciatic nerve) can cause pain.

The primary causes of complaints must be determined on an individual basis.

Are there professionals who are particularly affected? What should we take into consideration in the workplace?

Professions at risk are those that require lots of sitting and give little opportunity for variation in everyday movement patterns, for example typical desk-based office jobs. People who are frequently seriously stressed and placed under pressure by their jobs also meet one of the requirements that, in combination with other factors, can increase the risk.

In addition to weakening the gluteus maximus, the fascia network reacts to a lack of movement with poorly hydrated 'lubrication proteins'. This encourages solidification and additional collagen networks (cross-links), which further limit the capacity for adaptation and resistance.

Furthermore, the sitting position in particular leads to a reduced exchange of fluids and reduced removal of metabolic waste products, including those via the lymph system. This arises because of poor circulation limiting the supply of oxygen and nutrients to the myofascial tissue. Over time, nerve function can also be impaired, as a result of both undersupply and the constant pressure from sitting. Restrictive trouser folds in the groin area and crossed legs can also have an impact.

The following short, general tips are recommended for the workplace:

- Make sure your workplace is optimally adjusted for you.
- Change your sitting position regularly (dynamic sitting) and don't cross your legs.
- Take your wallet out of your back pocket.
- Take advantage of opportunities to go and talk to colleagues, rather than telephoning them.
- Use breaks actively, for example walk around the block in the fresh air.
- Try standing or even walking during meetings.
- Keep a glass of water on your desk, drink from it regularly and keep it topped up.
- Always take breaks of one to two minutes from sitting.
- Try some of the specific exercises in this book that can be easily integrated into your office routine.

Are there special tests that indicate piriformis syndrome?

You can use some simple tests to determine for yourself roughly how your piriformis muscle is doing, and whether you should consider any preventive measures. If it is tense and can no longer be loosened, it is in an upright position in relation to the thigh (to which it is attached) and often in an outer rotation. This can be seen very clearly if you look down and your foot points outwards rather than straight forwards. Is there a difference between your feet?

Another test you can do yourself is to cross your legs with the outer ankle resting on the other knee. If this causes painful tension in the buttocks, it is a possible sign. But, of course, this alone does not mean you definitely have piriformis syndrome.

The term *syndrome* always stands for a group of symptoms that we then identify as an illness. This means there are various signs that, when put together, lead to a diagnosis of piriformis syndrome. These signs primarily include the location, progression and characteristics of the pain. In our case, this is generally one-sided, deep-seated pain in the buttocks, which radiates into the back of the thigh to the knee and sometimes beyond. There may also be pain in the groin area.

There are also muscle length tests and muscle function tests that can be carried out for the piriformis muscle, as with other muscles. These tests enable doctors and therapists to quickly determine whether the muscle is 'shortened', and whether it can still cope with its intended movement function and power delivery. As a tense piriformis muscle can irritate other nerves in addition to the sciatic nerve, which can then in turn cause imbalances in other muscles in the buttocks and pelvis, tests for these affected muscles are also sensible. Furthermore, other causes that can lead to the same symptoms should be eliminated.

Are there similar conditions that are often confused with piriformis syndrome? Can the symptoms overlap?

Often an intervertebral disc protrusion or hernia is suspected, as the symptoms are very similar in terms of pain in the buttocks and leg. In this case, an MRI is carried out without delay, and the images will show whether there is actually damage to the intervertebral disc. This then confirms the suspicion.

However, we know from scientific studies and experience from unsuccessful operations that a protruding intervertebral disk with irritation of the nerve root is only responsible for the pain in a small number of cases. And even when this is the cause, the disk has been squeezed out by incorrect muscular tension – it isn't an independent creature that one day decided to leave the spinal column! This is why, in my opinion, myofascial tension should always be taken into account and compensated for (with the obvious exception of cauda equina syndrome, which is an emergency case). Experience shows that the treatment of this tension, in combination with specific exercises, is generally successful.

In addition to the well-known sciatic nerve, the pinching of other nerves in the buttocks as a result of muscle cramps or squeezing through narrowed spinal openings, particularly in the lower part (L5/S1) between the spine and the sacral bone, can also cause similar symptoms in the buttocks and leg.

An inflamed sacroiliac joint can also cause pain in the buttocks, but generally in the upper part. However, studies show that this can also radiate into the leg and even into the knee, which contradicts previous beliefs. Pain in the lower back relating to issues in the joints in the spine also acts in a similar way.

Furthermore, the piriformis muscle is connected to the organs known as *gonads* – the testicles and ovaries. As the nerves supplying this area come from the same segments of the spine, and these two elements can thus mutually influence each other, an organ issue can also be the primary cause.

Which test(s) do you recommend for checking for nerve root irritation? Is the straight-leg raise, for example, useful?

Yes, the straight-leg raise, with its several variations, is obviously the classic test. It consists of the doctor or therapist slowly raising your straight leg as you lie on your back. Depending on the angle at which pain occurs or gets worse, and depending on the characteristics of the pain, extension pain can be traced back to either the sciatic nerve or the muscles in the back of the thigh. If the pain in the affected leg is also triggered by lifting the straightened leg on the other side (cross straight-leg raise), nerve root irritation is likely.

Studies show that when the straight-leg raise test is positive (occurrence of pain in leg), the probability of nerve root involvement is high (91%); however, the contrary does not give such a clear conclusion – even if the test is negative, the nerve root may still be involved.

Further neurological tests are thus important if nerve root irritation is suspected, including testing for numbness, paralysis, loss of/reduced reflexes with weakness in the relevant reference muscle, and nerve conduction. With pure piriformis syndrome, the straight-leg raise test is generally negative.

Are there special trigger points that indicate piriformis syndrome?

By trigger points, we mean pain points that cause pain to be transmitted to other areas. When the piriformis muscle cramps up, there are generally two trigger points along its length: one is closer to the sacral bone, in the mid-buttock area, and the other is towards the head of the inner thigh, in the lower, outer quadrant of the buttocks. These are also used for establishing a diagnosis.

In addition, the aforementioned imbalances in other muscles in the buttocks and pelvis can cause further trigger points to appear, for example along the lower edge of the pelvic ridge and side hip areas.

Nevertheless, this must be observed in conjunction with other symptoms in order to diagnose piriformis syndrome.

Conventional medicine versus osteopathy for piriformis syndrome: which doctor can help?

I wouldn't say 'versus'. Ideally, they complement each other, and potentially other disciplines too.

The two techniques have fundamentally different approaches. Classic conventional medicine is symptom-based, divergent, localised medicine with drugs and operations to deal with pain directly, where it occurs. When the warning light comes on, the bulb is changed. The reason why the warning light is on is only looked into and handled in very few cases. In my opinion, conventional medicine has the most merit in acute situations, such as injuries.

In the case of piriformis syndrome, after a differential diagnosis by a sports doctor, orthopaedist and/or neurologist, I see little point in a conventional medicine approach, as the condition usually develops slowly. If extreme pain should occur, it can be helpful to fight this in the short-term with pain-relief medication or targeted injections. These numb the acute pain so that the patient is more relaxed, enabling the movement that is so important for tissue blood supply. Many wait too long, however, because they are satisfied with the initial relief of symptoms, thinking everything is fine again. But, of course, problems continue to simmer.

As my previous answers have made clear, it is necessary to go further and think of the body as an interconnected and interactive unit.

This is the approach of osteopathy as a holistic therapy method. We look for the causes, in other words the reason why the warning light is on; we then treat the whole system in its totality – the bones, muscles, fascia, organs, nervous system, etc. The body is then able to regulate itself. This leads to sustainable results.

How does stress affect piriformis syndrome on a day-to-day basis?

Stress is an issue with all illnesses, as it limits our ability to heal ourselves.

I always recommend a truly holistic approach. This means that when I talk about stress, I am referring not only to the stress we associate with time pressure – having too much to do and barely keeping up – but also to stress factors of any kind that our bodies have to deal with. These include emotional stress, noise, digital stress, exposure to radiation, environmental toxins, stress from poor nutrition, relentless exercise, basic attitude to life, and so on.

In all these examples, our bodies are in a state of alert. Our bodies produce stress hormones, such as adrenaline and cortisol, which cause our muscles and fascia to contract, particularly the pelvic floor and hip muscles. This means that we are constantly in a state of increased basic tension, and in most cases we do little to combat this.

Inevitably this leads to poorer blood circulation and reduced lymph flow, limiting nutrient and oxygen supply and the removal of waste products. Organ function is impaired, and the nervous, immune and endocrine systems are irritated. The result is that the whole body as a unit is affected.

What type of therapy do you recommend for acute piriformis syndrome?

If the diagnosis is certain, I combine physical therapy, primarily osteopathy and myofascial kinematics with special exercises that the patient can carry out at home or even at the office. I see patients accepting their individual responsibility as an essential component for a sustainable recovery.

My personal motto is: help people to help themselves. Clarifications on these stress factors, particularly those relating to nutrition and attitude, as well as support for making changes, are part of my holistic approach.

It is only when we observe our behaviour and thoughts and give our bodies the right stimuli, instead of bullying ourselves on a daily basis, that we can avoid the warning light coming on again in the near future.

How long does it take to see an improvement?

With pure piriformis syndrome, an initial improvement can often be felt very quickly, within one to three treatments. However, the time required for a complete recovery differs greatly from person to person, and is difficult to predict. Other than the existing duration of the syndrome and the circumstances, the period of recovery also depends on how willing the patient is to contribute, and can vary from a few weeks to a few months.

What role does the mobilisation and stabilisation of the hips/sacroiliac joint play with regard to piriformis syndrome?

A healthy, functional hip and pelvic area requires both stability and a certain level of mobility. In terms of the myofascial chains, this means that we should be aiming for a balanced myofascial situation, with no imbalances, throughout the whole body.

But which measures are needed for this must be decided on an individual basis. This is because, as already mentioned, there are various different causes of piriformis syndrome; often, however, there is a lack of stability.

Index

abduction, 63
acupuncture, 76
adductors, 47 *see also*: stretches for hip
    mobility
    stretch relieves hips, 48
ankle dorsiflexion test, 13

Baby camel stretch, 44
Baby cradle exercises, 31
Bragard's sign, 13
buttock muscles, 68–69
    bridge with mini-band, 71
    diagonal extension in tabletop
        position, 69
    knee bend exercise, 70

chair exercises, 39
    half chair half ankle to knee
        exercise, 40

    for hamstrings, 47
    for inner thighs, 50
    seated ankle on knee, 39
    thighs and psoas stretch, 43
cold treatment for nerve inflammation,
    76
combination exercise, 67
conscious movement as prevention, 80
    interconnected pain, 81–82
    movement diversity and quality, 80
    test for nerve root irritation, 85

diagonal extension exercise in tabletop
        position, 69
diet *see also*: inflammation; sleep
    impact on muscles, 18
    recommendation, 19

extension-related pain, 13

fascia, 51
    and back pain, 52
    roller, 52
    rolling speed, 52–53
forward fold exercise, 46
    with stacked legs, 32

gluteus maximus, 69

half chair half ankle to knee pose
        exercise, 36, 40
hamstring
    with chair exercise, 47
    tension, 45
heat treatment for muscle tension, 76
hip, 14
    flexor, 41

Iliotibial band syndrome (ITBS), 79
inflammation *see also*: diet
    promoters of, 18–19
    as response to injury, 18
injury response, 18
isometric exercise, 64

kinesiology taping, 77
knee
    bend on balance pad, 70
    down twist exercises, 27, 28
    to opposite shoulder exercise, 25

leg
    flexors exercise, 45
    knotting exercise, 26
localized stretches, 21, 23 *see also*:
        lying on back stretching;
        Seated stretching exercises

on both sides, 24
    duration of, 23
    passive stretching, 24
lower back pain, 16
lunge exercise, 42
lying butterfly exercise, 48
lying on back exercises, 24
    knee-down twist exercise, 27, 28
    knee to opposite shoulder exercise, 25
    leg knotting exercise, 26

mini-band, 66
muscle hardening, 18
muscles strengthening, 22, 58
    abduction, 63
    health effects of, 58
    outer rotation with abduction, 67–68
    progression with mini-band, 66
    recommendations for, 59
    seated press exercise, 64
    side lying with bent knee exercise, 62
    standing one-leg lift exercise, 65
    standing toes outward exercise, 60
    tabletop leg lift exercise, 63
    tree exercise, 61
myofascial relaxation, 21, 51

nerve root
    inflammation pain, 14
    irritation, test for, 85
NSAIDs (nonsteroidal anti-
        inflammatory drugs), 75

osteopathy, 76

pain
    in buttocks, 21

memory, 18
points for piriformis syndrome,
    85–86
promoters, 18–19
pain-relief, 75
    acupuncture, 76
    cold treatment for nerve
        inflammation, 76
    heat treatment for muscle tension,
        76
    kinesiology taping, 77
    NSAIDs, 75
    osteopathy, 76
    ultrasound therapy, 76
passive stretching, 24
Pfitzer, T., 80
Pigeon exercise, 34
piriformis muscle, 10, 16, 59 *see also*:
        muscles strengthening
    gluteus muscle and, 24
    psoas and, 44
    to reach, 25
    rolling with ball, 54
    rolling with roller, 55
piriformis syndrome, 9, 11, 16
        see also: conscious movement
        as prevention
    ankle dorsiflexion test, 13
    in athletes, 78, 79
    causes, 11, 15, 21–22
    diagnostic issues, 13, 84–85
    extension-related pain, 13
    hip mobilisation effect on, 88
    Iliotibial band syndrome, 79
    muscle strengthening, 22
    myofascial relaxation, 21
    nerve root inflammation pain, 14

    pain in buttocks, 21
    pain points for, 85–86
    professions at risk of, 82–83
    recommended therapy, 87
    repetitive stress, 15
    sports to be avoided in, 81
    straight-leg raise test, 13
    stress impact on, 87
    tests for, 83–84
    time for improvement, 88
    treatment options, 86
pressure on piriformis, 73

raising leg exercise, 47
repetitive stress, 15
revolved triangle exercise, 37–38
rolling with ball, 54
rolling with roller, 55
rotational exercises, 30
    knee-down twist exercises, 27, 28
    sitting half spinal twist exercises, 29
runner's knee, 79

sciatic nerve, 10
sciatic pain, 9
    common diagnoses, 12
seated exercises, 28
    ankle on knee exercise, 39
    Baby cradle exercises, 31
    forward fold with stacked legs
        exercises, 32
    Pigeon exercise, 34
    seated hurdle exercises, 33
    seated press exercise, 64
    Shoelace exercises, 30, 31
    sitting half spinal twist exercises, 29
side lying with bent knees exercise, 62

sitting, 72
 correct sitting technique, 73–74
 half spinal twist exercises, 29
 journal, 73
 pressure on piriformis, 73
 technique, 73–74
 variation of forward fold, 46
 variation of standing angle
  exercise, 50
sleep, 19–20 *see also*: diet
slipped disc, 16 *see also*: piriformis
  syndrome
standing exercises, 35
 half chair half ankle to knee
  pose, 36
 revolved triangle, 37–38
 standing angle exercise, 49
 standing at table exercise, 35
 standing one-leg lift exercise, 65
straight-leg lift, 45
 test, 13
stress effect, 17 *see also*: diet; sleep
 muscle hardening, 18
 for pain-free life, 20
 pain memory, 18

on physical and mental health, 17
stretches for hip mobility, 41
 Baby camel, 44
 forward fold, 46
 hamstrings with chair, 47
 hip flexor function, 41
 inner thighs with chair, 50
 leg flexors, 45
 lunge exercise, 42
 lying butterfly, 48
 raising leg, 47
 standing angle, 49, 50
 straight-leg lift, 45
 thighs and psoas stretch with
  chair, 43

tabletop leg lifts exercise, 63
thigh
 massage with roller, 56, 57
 and psoas stretch with chair, 43
traditional Chinese medicine (TCM),
  76
tree exercise, 61

ultrasound therapy, 76

About the Authors

Katharina Brinkmann is the founder of YOU Personal Training. In addition to being a yoga instructor and personal trainer, she is also a sports therapist. Among other things, her work focuses on fascia and mobility training, which she successfully combines in her book *Yoga – Fascia Training*.

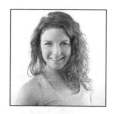

Nicolai Napolski is Editor in Chief of trainingsworld.com, the largest German portal for sports experts. An enthusiastic snowboarder, mountain biker and climber, he is no stranger to injuries! After several weeks of consulting doctors, he was diagnosed with piriformis syndrome by a physiotherapist. On realising that relatively little information was available on this topic, he was inspired to work with Katharina Brinkmann on this book.
No more buttock, leg or back pain!

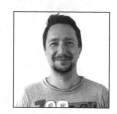

In her online programme, available at http://ischias-schmerzen.de/, Katharina Brinkmann shows you how you can easily and successfully treat yourself, in order to be pain-free in as little time as possible. Learn how you can use simple exercises and techniques to:

- Quickly stop acute pain
- Mobilise and strengthen your hips
- Easily handle trigger points yourself
- Sustainably build strength
- Return to a pain-free daily routine

Visit **http://ischias-schmerzen.de/** and gain the upper hand over your piriformis syndrome!

A Practitioner's Guide to Sacroiliac Joint Dysfunction and Piriformis Syndrome

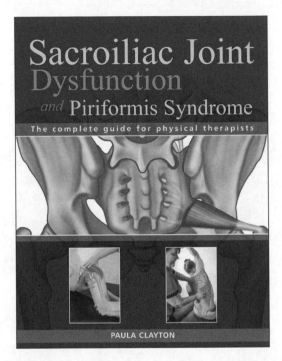

Applications for soft tissue therapy have increased significantly over the last decade. Perhaps the greatest area of growth has been around sports and caring for athletes. Multiple soft tissue, manipulative, and needling techniques have become mainstream tools in the therapist "tool box", whether aiding in athlete recovery, performance enhancement, or injury prevention.

Sacroiliac Joint Dysfunction and Piriformis Syndrome looks at dysfunction and injury, assessment, current understanding from the literature, and evidence-based treatment options at a therapist's disposal. This book offers the 'how' but more importantly the 'why', as to the map of approach one can take: if you cannot answer the WHY when beginning treatment, you shouldn't really attempt anything until you have an answer.

Clayton brings her years of expertise to this fully illustrated color guide, showing step-by-step how to correct dysfunction using a wide range of modalities.

colour, paperback